THE MEDICAL ENTREPRENEUR

PEARLS, PITFALLS & PRACTICAL BUSINESS ADVICE FOR DOCTORS

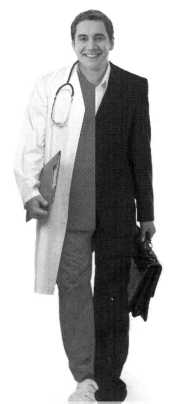

Steven M. Hacker, MD

www.TheMedicalEntrepreneur.com

Nano 2.0 Business Press

First Edition

Foreword written by Daniel M. Siegel, MD MS
(Management & Policy)

Nano 2.0 Business Press
Copyright © 2010 Steven M. Hacker MD
All rights reserved.

ISBN-10: 0615407137
EAN-13: 9780615407135
Library of Congress Control Number: 2010938047

REVIEWS FROM LEADING PHYSICIANS AND BUSINESS EXPERTS:

"We do not do enough to prepare our trainees for the business of practice. Likewise, so many creative physicians have commercializable ideas, but find out the hard way how a good idea does not a successful business make. Hacker's book is a gem in that it speaks to both of these challenges in an engaging way. It is chock-full of wisdom, easily read, and very enjoyable reading. I'll be recommending it to all of our trainees."
Joseph C. Kvedar, MD
Director, Center for Connected Health
Partners HealthCare System, Inc.
Associate Professor of Dermatology
Harvard Medical School

"After reading this book, I am now more certain than ever that my impressions of Dr. Hacker nearly twenty years ago were correct. His book is an honest, open, forthright attempt to share with his colleagues those precious details he has learned about establishing a medical practice and becoming an entrepreneur. I thought this book was fun to read, informative, concise, and blatantly honest. As I told Dr. Hacker after reading his book, 'I think you have taught an old dog some new tricks.' "
Franklin P. Flowers, MD
Professor, University of Florida College of Medicine
Department of Medicine, Division of Dermatology and Cutaneous Surgery

Excerpts from foreword written by Dr. Daniel Siegel

"Part I allows the reader to envision the necessary activities for opening his or her own practice in the voice of the author, while Part II is a guide for budding entrepreneurs. Part II covers victories and defeats in clear, concise tones that anyone can appreciate and empathize with.

Hemingwayesque, concise, and practical, this book would be an ideal gift from department chairs to their senior residents at the start of their last year of training, or a personal purchase around the same time if the chairperson is too cheap to buy it for you. If you are reading this, turn the page and take the roller-coaster ride. Enjoy!"

Daniel Mark Siegel MD, MS (Management and Policy)
Clinical Professor of Dermatology, SUNY Downstate
Director, Procedural Dermatology Fellowship
American Academy of Dermatology President Elect 2011

"Dr. Hacker's book effectively dispels the notion that 'doctors aren't good business people.' His personal example proves otherwise, and now his book can help other doctors break through that mold, too. Written with clear examples drawn from his experience, the book lays out—step by step—the tools and mind-set needed to create, launch, and profitably run a business. Kudos to the author."

Jeff Zbar
Author, Speaker, and Business Expert
ChiefHomeOfficer.com

FOREWORD
by Daniel Mark Siegel MD, MS

Steve Hacker is a neat guy. (If I thought he wasn't, I would not have agreed to write this foreword!).

In addition to being a real doc who sees patients in a private practice that he built from the ground up, he is a serial entrepreneur (unlike a serial killer who may dine on his victims, Steve can, as you will learn after reading the book, sometimes afford steak and lobster!) who has found a way to look at an unfilled niche in the business world and fill it in a profitable fashion.

In contrast to many of us who can simply connect the dots, he can wring money out of the dots and the lines between them that, in this regard, makes him more like Steve Jobs than you or me. In fact, Steve Hacker goes one up on Steve Jobs, as the latter has never been known to effectively treat skin cancer (though an app for that is rumored to available in the next version of the iPhone OS).

Despite the explosive growth of digital technologies, medical students, residents, and fellows still walk around with a soft-cover, often spiral-bound "manual" that is a concise, readable summary of the core techniques and knowledge of a particular specialty tucked into the pocket of their white coat. These white coats they wear have large pockets, as this little tome (I am assuming handbook sized or annotatable electronic, as a big, hardcover book such as *Surgery of the Skin: Procedural Dermatology*, by Robinson, Hanke, Siegel, and Fratila, does not fit in a pocket but should be bought anyway) will be a requirement for finishing trainees to have on hand, annotate, refer back to, and otherwise use as a road map to their first year in practice.

Part I, in the voice of the author, allows the reader to envision the necessary activities for opening his or her own practice, while Part II is a guide for budding entrepreneurs. Part II covers victories and defeats in clear, concise tones that anyone can appreciate and empathize with.

Hemingwayesque, concise, and practical, this book would be an ideal gift from department chairs to their senior residents at the start of their last year of training, or a personal purchase around the same time if the chairperson is too cheap to buy it for you. If you are reading this, turn the page and take the roller-coaster ride. Enjoy!

Daniel Mark Siegel MD, MS (Management and Policy)
Clinical Professor of Dermatology, SUNY Downstate
Director, Procedural Dermatology Fellowship
American Academy of Dermatology President Elect 2011

ACKNOWLEDGMENTS

I would like to thank the following people:

The loves of my life: my wife, Jill, and my children, Simon, Emily, and Elliot. Their enduring patience with all my crazy ideas, including the writing of this book, made everything possible.

My dad. He inspired me to be an entrepreneur.

Gary Lesnik and Craig Sterling, as the closest of friends since ten years of age, their encouragement and willingness to discuss my business ideas are what made many of them possible.

TABLE OF CONTENTS

SAVE THE DATE!
Earn CME hours and attend The Medical Entrepreneur Symposium March 29-April 1, 2012 at the Delray Beach Marriott Hotel in sunny south Florida.

RECEIVE CME CREDITS WHILE HEARING EXPERTS LECTURE ON EVERYTHING YOU NEED TO KNOW TO BE SUCCESSFUL IN PRACTICE AND AS A PHYSICIAN ENTREPRENEUR!

Register online at **www.TheMedicalEntrepreneur.com** and enter **coupon code TME2012** for additional 10% off registration fee.

IF AFTER READING THIS BOOK YOU WOULD LIKE TO...
Email the author questions or ask his advice for any issues concerning your medical practice or entrepreneurial venture, then try The Medical Entrepreneur Hotline. It is always available to help you with your business or medical practice. Visit www.TheMedicalEntrepreneur.com for details.

Want free practice updates and inside information on the latest trends and issues in medical practice from the author?
Email steven@stevenhacker.com with subject line "Updates"

YOU CAN BE A CARING DOCTOR AND A SAVVY BUSINESSPERSON

I am a doctor. I am an entrepreneur. I have spent the last fifteen years working both in private practice and in business. I have written this book because medical school does not prepare physicians for business. As doctors, we spend so much time learning about the human condition that we neglect to learn the basic fundamentals of running a business. The irony is that to practice medicine successfully today, a doctor must be equally as versed in the art of business as he or she is in the art of medicine.

A doctor can wear both hats. He or she can be both a caring physician and a savvy businessperson. This book steps in where no other book or course does for physicians.

As a physician in private practice, I bring a unique perspective that offers practical knowledge to doctors, young and experienced, who open the pages of this book. I have gone through the challenges of setting up my own solo practice. I set up my practice immediately out of residency. It became very successful and quickly grew to over twenty thousand patients.

At the same time I also built and sold two unrelated Internet-based technology businesses. As a "serial entrepreneur," I have started companies that have grown to become household names. The companies that I have started have gone on to serve millions of people and generate hundreds of millions of dollars in cumulative revenue over the last decade. While practicing medicine, I single-handedly negotiated deals with Fortune 500 companies, including Microsoft, Holland America Lines, L'Oreal, and more.

I have made several mistakes. I have had my failures. I write this book in the hopes of helping others avoid those mistakes. The lessons I learned from my mistakes as a businessman and physician are the basis for this book.

I have written this book in two parts.

This first part of this book is for all medical students, doctors entering private practice, young physicians that are in residency training programs, and experienced health care providers that are leaving a group practice to "go it alone." I write about the struggles I encountered and mistakes I made as I set up my own practice. I will detail the initial critical steps that every health care provider must take before seeing his or her first patient.

The second part of the book is for all health care providers, no matter their age or specialty, including those in academia, research, and private practice. It is not uncommon for academic or research-based physicians to want to commercialize their research or ideas. Since they have no experience in creating entrepreneurial ventures, this part of the book will help academic physicians better understand this process. Also, due to decreased reimbursements, many creative physicians in private practice want to supplement their incomes with entrepreneurial ventures. This part of the book explains what these doctors need to consider before launching any business. The second part of this book will teach an understanding of raising capital, negotiating contracts, hiring a management team, organizing corporate structure, delegating board seats, and more.

This is a business book for all health care providers regardless of their specialty. It is easy to use. Whenever relevant "real life" issues arise, doctors may quickly find how I dealt with a similar problem. I have identified critical points that must be remembered. I notate those sections with terms familiar to medical students and doctors, such as "Pearls" and "Pitfalls to Avoid." A pearl is a term that we used in medical school to refer to small facts about a condition that should be remembered. I annotate "Pearls" for those facts that I think you absolutely need to remember. I annotate "Pitfalls to Avoid" so you will not make costly mistakes as you set up your practice. Throughout the book, I have also included lists of action items on a variety of subjects. For your reference, I have designated these areas as "Tables".

I have also included unbiased expert opinions from attorneys on critical topics related to medicine or the business of medicine. I have identified these opinions as "Stat Consults" and separated them into easy to read textboxes. As a result, this book will provide you with instant access to expert legal opinions that would generally cost hundreds of dollars per hour if you were to ask an attorney the same question.

ACADEMIA OR PRIVATE PRACTICE?

Your first decision should be academia versus private practice. Academia is an incredible and inspiring career. It is different from private practice. Academia would include faculty positions at teaching institutions. The rewards of academia often are less tangible than the financial rewards of private practice. However, they are no less important. It is a personal decision. Teaching and research can provide exciting, engaging, and unique life opportunities. I wrestled with this decision throughout my residency training. For many reasons which I will discuss later I chose a career in private practice. The first section of the book is for those doctors, like myself, that have elected to enter private practice rather than academia.

IS PRIVATE PRACTICE STILL ALIVE AND WELL IN THE UNITED STATES?

Anyone that is a health care provider can go into private practice and be successful regardless of age, sex, race, and faith. You can be successful regardless of governmental health care reform. There will always be the opportunity to profit from your own practice.

The private practitioner is prototypical of the small American business. The private practitioner, no matter the political rhetoric, will always survive and thrive. We are the essence of small business in America. We are emblematic of the spirit of capitalism. And although corporate America wants to shut you down, acquire you, convert you, or push you into a large group, as long as capitalism survives in America, you will not only survive, you will succeed.

Initially it may be intimidating, but don't allow it. Anyone, even without any formal business education or experience, can start his or her own practice.

In most situations, you will make more money than you would in a group practice. You will have freedom, individual creativity, and lifestyle benefits. You will create your own rules and your own hours. You will answer to no one. Going it on your own is exciting, liberating, and rewarding. So, don't hesitate! You will not regret it.

Everyone that I have ever spoken to, encouraged, or helped to go into solo private practice has achieved personal and financial success beyond their expectations.

I have never met a single doctor who has started his or her own practice and regretted it. Have the "guts" to do it! You and your family will be grateful.

WHAT DO YOU DO WITH A GREAT IDEA?

Part II of this book is for you, the creative doctor, in private practice or academia, young or old, who has the desire to create another business and become an entrepreneur. If you have a great idea or a creative urge to try another business, then this section is a must read. If, like many other doctors, you are looking for additional sources of income or are inspired to have a side business, then my experiences will help you avoid making the same mistakes that I made. If you are in academia and would like to commercialize your research, then this section will help you understand how to create that business.

In medical school we are not prepared for business. We are not taught how to raise capital. We are not taught about the business owner or founder's liabilities and the implications of raising capital. We do not learn about "burn rates," "dilution," "board seats," "options," and "angel investors." We are given no books to read about venture capitalists, trademark protection, patent protection, online commerce, and Web development. We are not schooled in executive management, organization charts, and sales and marketing teams. We are not given courses on negotiating contracts and leases.

I have founded ten corporations in the last fifteen years while practicing medicine. My experience in raising capital and selling these companies is invaluable for health care providers. I am excited to share my stories with you and, most importantly, point out the mistakes I made and successes I had. This part of the book will provide you with real-life advice based upon the incredible ups and downs I have had as a medical entrepreneur.

PART I:

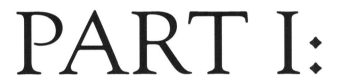

Everything you need to know before you see your first patient

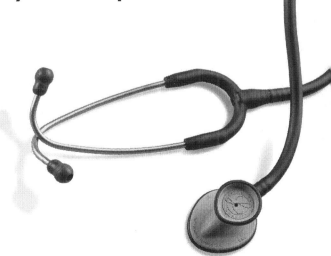

CONGRATS, YOU'RE A DOCTOR, NOW HOW DO YOU MAKE MONEY?

I remember the time I was a senior resident. It was the beginning of my final year of postgraduate training. I knew I had decisions to make. I was conflicted. Would I go into academics or would I go into private practice? This was the first question I needed to answer. Throughout medical school and residency, the allure of academics and the urging of my professors had led me down the path of academics. The collegiality and sense of purpose with academics made this a difficult choice for me. I did not want to disappoint my professors. However, I wanted to get into private practice. Honestly, I wanted to make some money. It had been a long haul, and twelve years of education and training had brought me to this juncture. I had no debt, thankfully. I had no money either.

My biggest concern was the same concern that many residents had: if I chose private practice, would my professors consider me a sellout? If I did not join them in academics, would their disappointment affect my ability to get a competitive job in private practice? I knew I needed their letters of recommendation to get a position after residency. I was nervous when I finally decided that I would go into private practice. I had to tell the faculty that I would not be entering academics. I was hesitant to let them know that I would be looking for a job during my senior year of residency.

It turns out, after speaking to many residents, that these trepidations are common. Many during residency share them. However, these concerns are unfounded. The faculty are aware of and understand your situation. They are eager to help you get a job after graduation. Teachers know you must begin looking for work. You may feel like you are betraying an unspoken code of commitment to academia. You are not. Planning for private practice should begin in your senior year of residency. And, if you are going to set up your own solo practice, then you must start at least ten to twelve months before you see your first patient.

Once you have decided to make the leap into private practice, you must decide if you are going to join a group practice or set up a solo practice. I wrestled with this decision for some time. At first I thought I was better suited joining a group practice. I knew I had no private practice experience. I was worried because I didn't understand medical billing. I was concerned that I might need "backup" if I didn't know how to treat a patient. I didn't think patients would want to come see me as their doctor. It is easy to understand why most people choose group practices over a solo practice. These concerns and fears are universal. They are also completely unfounded.

Nevertheless, I went down the path of joining a group practice. I interviewed with several groups. Each group had a different personality. In selecting a group practice, I had defined my own set of criteria: the doctors had to practice medicine ethically, they had to be well respected, and the physicians had to tolerate various personality types. A group practice is like a marriage, and if there are personalities that conflict with your own, the odds are overwhelming that you will not be happy in that practice.

The experiences I had while interviewing were interesting. I won't forget the time a senior partner of a large, well-known practice went out of his way to let me know that all the doctors in the group were expected to attend the same church. Although these were a nice bunch of guys, that was a red flag. It was too coercive and personal for my comfort.

The one group I liked the best happened to be the most successful and most respected group in our area. They entertained my wife and me with a very expensive dinner. All the partners were there. I was impressed. I felt that this group was an ideal fit for my personality. I was told that partnership would be offered. However, after I received the contract offer in writing, the details of the partnership and compensation were lower than I expected. It appeared that I would generate hundreds of thousands of dollars in revenue for their practice. I would only receive a fraction of the revenue collected. I would work for three to four years before becoming a partner. Partnership meant that I would be able to keep what I collected minus the cost of overhead. And yet, the overhead expenses included, amongst other things, rent in the building that some of the partners owned. The discrepancy in my income as compared to the amount of revenue I generated was so great that it prompted me to consider other options.

Solo practice was one of these options. I modeled out what I thought I could generate on my own in solo private practice. I accounted for seeing only a few patients at first. I still would make more money than I would if I joined the group practice. I realized that it did not make sense for me to join the most alluring, most well respected practice in our area. I politely sent a letter thanking the practice for my offer and their time. I committed myself to learning everything I could about starting my own practice. Ironically, that same group practice split up over the ensuing few years due to partner disagreements.

The lesson learned here is, don't be influenced by the "glitz and glamour" (what I call "sex appeal") of another practice. Analyze objectively, not emotionally, the offer you receive before accepting it. Do not get seduced by the practice size and appearance. I often advise senior residents to not sign an employee contract with any group practice the first year or two. Be an independent contractor and work part-time for a few different practices. You may spend two days a week with one practice and three days a week with another. You will learn all you need to about yourself and the practice in that time period. You will see if there are any "warts" in the practice. You will avoid contractual problems in the event the practice is not right for you. It is very common for doctors to sign an employee contract, join the wrong practice and regret their decision later.

If you are set on joining a group practice, make sure you understand the revenue model for owners, partners, associates and employees. Calculate the precise amounts you will make for the practice and make for yourself. You can estimate how much revenue you will earn by understanding how many patients you will be seeing per day. Multiply that number by the average amount billed or the average amount collected per patient. Subtract the overhead percentage from that total amount. That is what is left over for you and the practice. These numbers are readily available. The partners in the practice can provide them for you. In order for this to be an accurate estimate, the amounts must be relevant for the type of practice you will have. In other words, if you will be mostly surgical or medical, then the respective fees projected should reflect that. Understand what "partnership" means. If, as a partner, you have to pay overhead to other partners, then be cautious. Make sure you ask about "common" revenue earned and shared. For instance, lab revenue generated from the practice is considered common revenue. Find out how you share in that revenue as either a partner or employee. Go through the exercise of analyzing amount collected versus amount received with any group practice offer. You will find more often than not that you will make more money on your own than in the group practice. The reason is simple. The group practice must make a percentage of the revenue you generate. The amount that it makes from your work will be the extra amount you would keep for yourself if you went into solo practice. Aside from income issues, some specialists feel that they must join a group practice due to call and hospital coverage. However, now there are many "hospitalists" and other soloists that share call or provide hospital inpatient coverage with each other. The burden of call and cross coverage is much easier to overcome today than it was years ago. So, don't worry about that.

You will earn more money in solo practice, have more personal freedoms, and be your own boss. It is a no-brainer. You must go out on your own. And you must get started as soon as possible.

FIRST STEP, SET UP A CORPORATION

There are many theories about picking a name for your practice. You can pick a name that uses your real name and is very professional, such as John Doe, MDPA.

You can be creative and give your practice a fictional name, such as "Palm Beach Medical Institute." You can do both. Use one as a corporate name registered with the state. Use the other name as a "D/B/A" (Doing Business As) name.

Years ago people would create a name for the business starting with an A. The purpose of this strategy would be so the business would be listed first in the Yellow Pages. For instance, my practice name was Advanced Dermatologic Care and Cancer Center. Fifteen years ago, I was listed first under "Dermatologists" in the Yellow Pages. The Internet is now more important than the Yellow Pages for advertising. Sophisticated search engines utilize complex search algorithms to populate search returns. This makes having an A to start your practice name obsolete. Sites do not get listed on search engines in alphabetical order.

The name of your business should be short. It should be easy to remember so patients can easily recall your Web site. The name itself may include common search terms or common keywords. Terms should be relevant to your practice.

PITFALLS TO AVOID

Don't make the mistake of selecting a practice name or corporation name until you have verified and purchased a matching Internet domain name.

The Internet domain name is the URL (Universal Resource Locator) or the Web address of your Web site. You should have a Web site domain name that matches your practice name. Make sure your domain name is available on the Internet. This is easy to check by visiting sites such as Network Solutions or GoDaddy.com. You can search these sites and buy the domain name that closely matches your practice name.

You need to decide what type of corporation you will be forming. Businesses incorporate for many reasons, including tax advantages and debt and liability protection. In the event of a lawsuit, it is difficult for lawyers to puncture the "corporate veil" of a corporation. The corporate veil will protect your personal assets from debt or liabilities associated with the corporation.

There are a few different corporation types to choose from. Each structure has tax implications and liability implications. The corporation types that you may choose from are subchapter C corporations (C corps), subchapter S corporations (S corps) and Limited Liability Corporations (LLCs). The S corporation rules are contained in subchapter S of Chapter 1 of the Internal Revenue Code (sections 1361 through 1379). A C corporation is a corporation in the United States that, for federal income tax purposes, is taxed under 26 U.S.C. § 11 and Subchapter C (26 U.S.C. § 301 et seq.) of Chapter 1 of the Internal Revenue Code.

When I first was setting up my practice, I had no idea of the differences between corporation types. I relied completely on my accountant. In hindsight, he was not the best person for the job. He was what I call a "schmoozer." He spent more time asking me personal questions about my family then he did actually working on my accounting. He was "too" friendly. He would try to impress me by remembering the ages and birthdates of my children. Yet he couldn't remember to file my returns on a timely basis. He was routinely missing filing deadlines or details related to comprehensive tax planning. A good accountant can be great, while a bad accountant can be disastrous. I have gone through four accountants in fifteen years. The last one is finally the one I want to have.

Initially we set up my practice as a C corporation. Although not wrong, it certainly created extra work. Every year we had to pay attention to income and expenses to avoid double taxations. Subsequently, I went through a series of accountants. All of them suggested I convert to an S corporation. I eventually did convert from a C to an S corporation. I was warned that if I sold my practice within ten years of converting from a C to an S corporation, I would still be taxed and potentially double taxed as a C corporation. Double taxation occurs when a corporate entity is taxed at both the corporate level (if the company shows profits at the end of the year) and then again at the individual level (personal income).

There are differences between corporation elections (types) that are important to understand. You should understand these differences so you can elect the most appropriate for your situation.

PEARL

Some advantages of S corporation:

1. Avoidance of double taxation.

2. Savings on payroll taxes via shareholder (owners of the company) distributions.

3. Taxes may be less on sale of practice if S corporation.

4. Income passes through to individual shareholder.

A C corporation carries the risk of "double taxation," or tax on corporate income and on distribution of dividends to stockholders. In a subchapter S corporation, all the profits pass through to the shareholders' (owners' of the company) individual tax returns. This means that shareholders only pay taxes on these profits through their personal tax returns. This is similar for sole proprietorships and LLCs (limited liability corporations). In summary, the S corporation itself does not pay income tax. It is often the easiest election for a doctor to manage.

PEARL

Some of the requirements of an S corporation election are:

1. Each S corporation shareholder must be a U.S. citizen or resident.

2. The S corporation can never have more than seventy-five shareholders.

3. S corporation profits or losses must be allocated in direct proportion to ownership interests. For example, if you only own 10 percent of a business, then you can only claim 10 percent of the amount lost or earned from that business on your personal income tax.

4. S corporations may not deduct the cost of fringe benefits provided to employee-shareholders that own more than 2 percent of the corporation.

PITFALLS TO AVOID

If you break any of these S corporation rules, you will be forced to be reclassified as a subchapter C corporation. This reclassification may subject you to additional taxes and penalties. You will lose all the S corporation benefits.

Once you have decided on the corporation name and elected a corporation type (i.e., S corp or C corp), you will need to write the articles of incorporation and corporate bylaws and create a board of directors. You will need the help of a corporate attorney for this. At this point, you will need to file and register your corporation with the state so that you can issue stock to shareholders. In a medical practice, you are usually the sole shareholder.

Don't let these steps intimidate you. They are mostly boilerplate processes. Attorneys will do the work for you. There are "do it yourself" Web sites and forms for this. However, the few dollars an attorney charges are worth it. This will ensure that the setup process is done right from the outset.

STAT CONSULT FROM JOHN IGOE, A CORPORATE ATTORNEY

Everyone is entitled to conduct business through a corporate entity to avoid personal liability for obligations to vendors and other creditors. Doctors should take advantage of this and avoid operating as sole proprietors. However, doctors, like other regulated professionals, cannot avoid liability for malpractice by operating as a corporation or LLC. Any practicing doctor should investigate the pros and cons of acquiring malpractice insurance.

In a profitable S corporation, you will have the ability to allocate profits between your salary, subject to withholding taxes, and dividends, subject only to ordinary income tax rates applicable to dividends, generally lower than the withholding tax burden. The IRS may review this allocation and insist on payment of "reasonable" salaries. As an obvious example, you would not pay yourself a salary of $10,000 and distribute profits as a dividend distribution of $500,000. If you demonstrate consistency with salary and bonus payments, you can save some taxes by distributing a portion of your profits as dividends. Consult your tax accountant on this issue. If you have other partners or investors in your business, dividends must be distributed to them on a pro rata basis, tied to ownership of shares in your company.

NEXT, TRADEMARK YOUR PRACTICE NAME

After you have filed formal paperwork with the state for your corporation and purchased a matching domain for your Web site, you can trademark the name. This is something you can do by yourself. It is very easy. You can trademark the name at www.uspto.org. If an attorney is already preparing your corporation documents, you could also ask him or her to trademark your business name, too. Ask him or her to do this for the amount of the filing fee ($275-$300) since he is already doing other work for you.

The first use of your trademark, as it is called, a common law trademark, may offer enough protection without officially registering the trademark. Common law trademark is defensible, but probably not as defensible as a registered trademark. Registering a trademark online is inexpensive. It may costs less than $300 if you do it yourself online. If your name is original and you fear someone might steal it, then trademark it. I register my trademarks online without the help of an attorney.

STAT CONSULT FROM HOWARD M. GITTEN, INTELLECTUAL PROPERTY ATTORNEY

TRADEMARKS

What Are They?

Trademarks protect the goodwill of your company. They in effect identify your company as the source of certain goods of a certain quality. A trademark is any word, name, symbol, or device used to identify the source or origin of products or services and to distinguish those products or services from others. When you hear McDonald's, it has a different connotation in your mind than Burger King, even for very similar products. You, as a consumer, know what to expect when you eat at McDonald's. Now think how confusing it will be and how upset McDonald's would be if Burger King changed the name of its famous burger to the McWhopper.

Everyone knows that words such as Sprite soda, Corvette convertible, and Google searches are valid and appropriate use of trademarks. It is also well known that numbers and letters have become very famous trademarks, such as BMW, 3M, and 1-800-FLOWERS as sources of goods and services; and, lastly, designs and logos also have great power as trademarks. Think of the Nike swoosh, Adidas stripes, Starbucks mermaid; all very strong trademarks in the mind of the consumer.

However, less conventional identifiers can also be used as trademarks. For example, sounds such as the roar of the MGM lion, the opening notes of Microsoft software, and even an attempt to trademark the Harley-Davidson engine sound. Fragrances such as stationery treated with a special fragrance can be trademarks. Shapes such as the unique shape of the Apple iPod or Lego building blocks have been given trademark protection. Colors such as the brown for UPS, Nexium's purple pill, and the distinctive pink, blue, and yellow artificial sweetener packets have all been used to establish brand awareness. I am sure that each of you, when reading this, have already identified the owners of the respective artificial sweetener colors; that is the ultimate test as to whether something has become a trademark. Lastly, the overall look, the trade dress, has been given trademark protection. For example, a distinctive décor and layout for most franchise restau rants, such as Hooters' orange and white uniforms and wooden décor or Chipotle's accent colors, metal, and wood, would be given trademark protection.

The government, in effect, is giving you a monopoly over a word and its use in commerce. So, like patents, there are certain hurdles which must be overcome in order to establish the strength and validity of your trademark. Words may be generic, descriptive, suggestive, or fanciful. Where your proposed trademark lies on that spectrum will govern the strength of its use as a trademark. By way of example, if you are a farmer and you wish to brand your new red, shiny fruit APPLE, the government will not grant you trademark rights because "apple" is generic for the red, shiny fruit. What would other farmers call their red, shiny fruit?

Similarly, if you are a baker and you wish to trademark your cakes and cookies which taste like the red, shiny fruit, whether they include the red, shiny fruit or artificial ingredients, as APPLE cookies you will not be allowed to enforce monopoly rights in that brand either. Such use is descriptive. How would other bakeries describe their apple-flavored products? Therefore, descriptive marks are, for the most part, not enforceable.

However, if you are manufacturing a perfume which smells sweet or fruity and wish to brand that perfume APPLE perfume, then the word is only suggestive of a characteristic of the product, and you will most likely be entitled to trademark protection. Better yet, if you are starting a computer company and name your product line APPLE, then this is fanciful and a strong mark.

However, words can change their status, and the spectrum discussed above is only a general yardstick. History is littered with examples of marks across the spectrum, including famous marks which have become generic. Generic marks such as "aspirin" and" thermos" both began as fanciful marks; Movie Channel or Healthy Choice may be considered descriptive bordering on suggestive marks. Suggestive marks are marks such as Priceline.com, and fanciful marks are marks like Kodak and Windows.

There are other rules as to which types of marks are not acceptable for protection even if fanciful. Immoral or scandalous matter, such as curse words, will most likely not be granted trademark protection. Deceptive matter such as "Fresh Florida Oranges" for oranges grown in California, or anywhere other than Florida, will not be granted protection. Lastly, surnames such as Anderson or Smith or famous names such as Johnny Carson can't be trademarked unless you are that person or the person is fictitious.

How Do I Get Mine?

Unlike a patent, which must be issued by the government, you do not need the government to obtain a trademark right. There are registered trademarks, those which have ® as an indicator of government issuance, and common law trademarks, indicated by the ™ symbol. Both are valid marks. The government grants the trademark rights in the registered ® trademark. Common law trademark (TM) rights develop over time with use in commerce until they become so famous that they have meaning in the general public as being from a single source.

The process for obtaining a trademark always begins with selecting an appropriate mark; one that is not scandalous, deceptive, descriptive, or generic. Then a trademark search should be performed to make sure that the mark is free for use and that you are not infringing the rights of others. This can be done by consulting an attorney, or at least preliminarily conducting an Internet word search or a search at USPTO.gov, where all pending and currently registered trademarks can be searched. Once you have cleared the mark, the rights in the trademark are created either through extensive commercial use, including advertising and promotion of the brand embodied by the trademark, or by filing with the government for registration.

Similar to the patent process, the trademark registration process begins with an application in which you identify the name or any special artwork associated with the word, such as a logo and a description of the goods and services being provided under that brand. Again, there are buildings full of examiners who determine first whether the word is appropriate to be a trademark and then make sure that it does not cause a likelihood of confusion with any other pending or registered mark (registrations of similar words for similar goods). It should be noted that as part of the government process, the government only screens marks in its system when determining a likelihood of confusion. However, it may look outside of the U.S. Patent and Trademark Office to determine whether or not a mark is deceptive, profane, generic, or descriptive.

What Good Are They?

Once trademark rights are established, they are rights to prevent others from using words in a manner which is confusingly similar to the way in which you use your trademark. Trademark infringement occurs when there is a likelihood of confusion between someone else's uses of a word (not necessarily the identical word) in a confusing manner. At the heart of the test is (1) a determination of how close in sound and connotation to the actual trademarks the words are; (2) how close the goods associated with each word are; (3) what the overlap is in the channels of trade for the goods covered by the competing trademarks; and (4) how smart the customers are for the respective goods. By way of example, there is a very small likelihood of confusion between Cadillac automobiles and Cadillac dog food. However, if Coors started selling Coke beer, then Coca Cola, the soda company, would most likely be suing the beer company. Like patents, these rights can be used to stop others from infringing your trademarks, or as a way to license others to use your brand with similar or even different goods.

STAT CONSULT FROM JOHN IGOE, CORPORATE ATTORNEY

Google is very thorough, but understand that Internet searches and reviews of public databases are not exhaustive. Someone may have established but unregistered common law rights to a trademark you want to use. It should not be a problem if you are in different lines of business, but official trademark searches, while more expensive, are much more comprehensive. This may not be necessary for your local practice.

NEXT, YOU WILL NEED A LINE OF A CREDIT AND A TEAM OF PROFESSIONALS SUCH AS ACCOUNTANTS, LAWYERS, AND INSURANCE AGENTS

A line of credit is your lifeline. It is the blood supply of your practice. The line of credit is what enables you to start your practice at anytime. It enables you to have cash flow while the practice grows. Almost all growing and profitable businesses have a line of credit. Your practice should be no different. The line of credit is what you use to pay yourself until you start generating sufficient revenue. The line of credit will help you to develop and grow your practice. It will allow you to make special equipment purchases when you want to and not only when you have the cash avail- able. This is critically important for any business. Medicine is no different. It is common to have slow periods of cash flow.

Cash flow can be an unpredictable variable. It may be unrelated to your charges. You may think you are doing great, seeing many patients, and generating significant charges. However, this does not equate to cash flow for your practice. Cash flow is related to payments received. Insurance com- panies and Medicare may, for whatever reason, hold your payments at different time periods. For instance, Medicare may hold payments when Congress debates over physician compensation. Medicare rates are set by Congress. These rates are subject to politics. Each year for the last few years, Congress has enacted payment changes to physician reimbursement. It has passed legislation to delay decreases in physician compensation, or it has passed legislation to decrease physician compensation. You may need the busi- ness line of credit to pay employees from time to time to protect you against unexpected decreases in cash flow.

Most banks are willing to give you a line of credit based upon your earnings potential. You may be able to "shop" the banks for a line of credit. Select the bank that offers the lowest interest rate and the lowest fees. Lines of credit renew annually or biannually. The banks may or may not charge a fee associated with each annual renewal. Many banks have a specialty division just for lending to physicians.

If a bank declines you credit, there are alternative financing options. Federal and state programs may be available, such as through the Small Business Administration (SBA) guaranteed loan program. If you are still unable to secure credit, then consider home equity financing. Additionally, the use of credit cards and equipment leasing may be viable short-term alternatives. Credit card financing can be costly, so I would suggest this only if you cannot find alternative financing. Credit card interest rates are high and burdensome. You should not carry credit card debt for more than thirty days.

Surround yourself with a reputable and reliable team of professionals. This includes an accountant, insurance agent, health care attorney, and corporate attorney. Speak with other doctors to find out whom they recommend.

STAT CONSULT FROM JEFF COHEN, BOARD-CERTIFIED HEALTH CARE ATTORNEY

Hiring a Lawyer

This is simple and common sense, since everyone hires consultants for a variety of things—from plumbing to accounting. Too often, doctors hire lawyers who don't have the relevant experience. Law, like medicine, has become super specialized. Just like you would not ask a gastroenterologist to handle a knee replacement, you ought to make sure the lawyer you choose has plenty of experience doing exactly what you need done. Even board certification (in Florida only, so far) may not mean the lawyer has the relevant experience. Ask!

The two bottom lines here are: (1) Hire someone with the experience necessary to get the job done. How many of the sorts of issues involving you has the lawyer dealt with? Does he or she have to do extensive research to learn the area of law or just to update the current status of the issue?; and (2) Get a clear agreement about price. A lawyer with the right experience regarding your issue will, at best, be able to give you a flat fee, and, at least, be able to give you a binding range of fees for (a) reviewing a document, (b) preparing one, and (c) finding an answer to your legal question. Certain things, however, like negotiating a contract, are nearly impossible to estimate.

When you ask about fees, try looking at it as though the lawyer is a plumber. Any lawyer with enough experience of the kind you need should be able to tell you: (1) what he or she will charge to prepare a document or to review one and give you comments, and (2) how long he or she thinks negotiation will take and how much it may cost. Some lawyers will agree to flat fees and also will agree to cap their fees.

A good accountant is critical. Do not think of your accountant as someone that just prepares your tax returns. You should have a dynamic relationship with your accountant. Seek his or her advice before making equipment purchases. Understand which purchases can be expensed and which will be capitalized. A capitalized expense may be one that has to be "booked" over several years. This means that you cannot fully expense it off your income in the year it was purchased. Expenses reduce your income and consequently affect the total income tax you pay. Purchases for consumables or salaries paid are examples of expenses that are fully realized in the year that are spent. You should work with your accountant to understand these and many other income and balance sheet principles.

You should negotiate fees with the accountant. Some accountants will charge you a monthly fee while others will charge you a fee at the end of the year. You should define their responsibilities. You should have a mutual understanding of the services that they will provide.

A good insurance agent will provide you with many alternatives. You will need to insure your practice, yourself, and your family. Insurance is for the unpredictable events in life. You should evaluate disability insurance options. Disability policies may be written that are job specific. You can insure yourself for the most profitable services you perform, e.g., surgery (if you are a surgeon). In the event something happens to your hands, for instance, you may continue to practice, but you can't do surgery. You should have insurance to cover for this.

Additionally, you should evaluate business interruption insurance to cover your practice expenses, such as payroll, in the event something happens to temporarily shut down your business. Business interruption insurance is important to keep your employees paid while you undergo an unexpected catastrophe with your office.

Office overhead insurance is another form of insurance that pays every employee but you in the event of a short-term disability or hospitalization. This can be helpful to retain key employees in the event you are disabled and cannot generate revenue.

Umbrella liability insurance is the insurance that covers your personal liability after your basic home and automobile liability coverage has stopped. This insurance is not related to your professional services coverage with malpractice. This insurance is personal liability for accidents that may occur outside of the office. Physicians are targets for lawyers in all aspects of life. An umbrella policy provides an extra layer of coverage on top of your other personal liability coverages.

Lastly, evaluate life insurance options: term versus universal versus whole life. Term is more affordable initially. Whole life is more expensive but provides a "cash value" portion to the policy that may be used for retirement planning. A traditional term life insurance policy covers you for a specified term. Premiums are fixed and often the most affordable. Term is ideal to provide protection for a limited time, such as to protect a mortgage. Variable life permanent insurance policies offer fixed premiums, but, unlike whole life, the policy does not build up cash value. Variable universal life permanent offers flexible premiums based upon the performance of the investments of the underlying policy. These policies are more risky because the investments may drop in value. As a result, the insured would see fewer death benefits and less cash value. I have both term and whole life policies. I purchased my term policies when I had no money, had two children, and had just finished residency. I purchased whole life later on. I would recommend that you discuss these options with your insurance agent.

The best time for estate planning and protection is now. As you consider life insurance, you need to consider irrevocable trusts and estate planning. Proper estate planning from the start will include wills, trusts, and various other measures to protect your assets and your beneficiaries from unnecessary taxes and lawsuits. Plan now rather than later. You need to have a trusted estate attorney advise you based upon active federal and state laws.

STAT CONSULT FROM KENNETH EDELMAN, AN ESTATE ATTORNEY

I have a few recommendations for doctors graduating from medical school and beginning to pursue their medical careers. These recommendations are practical advice for doctors in initiating their estate planning, which will last the balance of their lives.

Interview attorneys for different areas of need. You may need a corporate attorney to set up your practice, and you should seek an attorney who specializes in medical practices. You should find an estate planning attorney at an early age to set up your and your spouse's wills (and possibly trusts); this is a relationship that should last many years, and you need to seek an attorney who is compatible with you and your spouse, one who understands your situation. You and your spouse should both be present for the interview. Further, in case of potential malpractice litigation, you should find a malpractice defense attorney before any litigation is on the horizon, so that you are in position to act if necessary.

You should make sure that you understand everything that the attorney says to you. Don't just nod your head and make believe that you understand. And don't sign any document before fully comprehending what it does and its effects on your life and the lives of your children.

You (and your spouse) must have wills. In this way, you can each provide a mechanism for passing your assets *to each other, then your children (and grandchildren), at the lowest tax cost, and also protect your assets to the maximum extent possible.*

Proper estate tax planning generally requires the use of each spouse's estate tax "exemption." This is the amount that can pass estate-tax free (for federal tax purposes) at a person's death. In 2009, this amount was $3,500,000; so a married couple could potentially avoid estate taxation on up to $7,000,000, with full use of both spouses' exemptions. This year, 2010, there is currently no federal estate tax. In 2011 the exemption is due to decrease to $1,000,000 (although, as of this writing, there is a likelihood that the amount will be increased substantially, possibly back to $3,500,000).

Generally, for a married couple, use of each spouse's exemption is accomplished through the use of a trust, created by the first spouse at his or her death, for the use of the surviving spouse for his or her life. The amount funding this trust is equal to the exemption in effect at the first spouse's death (for example, in 2009, the amount would have been $3,500,000). On the surviving spouse's death, the assets in the trust, in addition to the amount of the surviving spouse's exemption, will pass estate-tax free to the children and/or grandchildren.

These days, when the estate tax law and the estate tax exemption are fluctuating, a typical will mechanism involves the use of a "disclaimer trust." A disclaimer is a document that, for estate tax purposes, has the effect of deeming the person making the disclaimer to have predeceased the decedent as to all or a portion of the estate. There is a great deal of planning that can be done with disclaimers, either to help fix a bad plan, or to make a good plan better. A <u>disclaimer document must generally be filed with the appropriate person within nine months after the decedent's death.</u>

For example, suppose that a doctor's will provides that all assets pass outright to her husband at her death. Suppose also that the will provides that if the husband files a disclaimer as to all or a portion of the estate, the portion that is disclaimed (not taken outright) passes to a trust for the husband. By passing to a trust for the husband, and ultimately to the descendants, the family can make use of the deceased wife's estate tax exemption. In addition, on the husband's death, the family can make use of his estate tax exemption. Therefore, the family will potentially avoid estate tax on an amount equal to both spouse's exemptions. However, if the total combined estate is small, or the exemptions in effect are extremely large, the husband may decide not to disclaim any portion of the wife's estate (thereby taking all assets outright, rather than in trust), which is simpler.

There are various trust mechanisms that may make sense for you and your family. Under a trust, which can be incorporated into a will, a third party (typically) will manage assets for the benefit of a family member. This can be beneficial taxwise, as well as asset-protection-wise. For example, suppose that your spouse dies and leaves his or her assets outright to you (or they pass to you via a joint account). Suppose also that there is an outstanding judgment against you. The judgment is enforceable against those inherited assets. However, if your spouse had left you the assets in a trust for your benefit, rather than outright, *the assets would not be available to the judgment creditors. Therefore, a trust, if properly drafted (for example, to include "spendthrift" language, which has the general effect of barring creditors), can provide tremendous protection against creditors.*

A trust can also be beneficial to protect assets passing to children or grandchildren from a bad marriage, lawsuits, or the child's own inability to handle money. Suppose your son has drug or alcohol issues, or enters a profession where he has significant potential for liability (such as medicine). A trust can protect those assets from your son himself or from third-party creditors. By naming a trustee whom you trust to manage the trust assets, and by giving that trustee direction as to how to manage those assets for your son's benefit, you can effectively control the assets and make sure that they are protected in the best way possible.

You can include in the trust any language that you want the trustee to consider, such as providing for tuition, travel to and from school, vocational training, trips to Europe, etc. In addition, you can provide for incentives for the child; for example, the trustee can make distributions to the child to match his or her wages, or wages above a set amount.

One type of trust, an irrevocable life insurance trust (or "ILIT"), is often used for life insurance. By purchasing a life insurance policy through an irrevocable trust, and making the trust the beneficiary of the policy, the proceeds at your death can avoid all estate taxation. Otherwise, the proceeds will be considered your assets, and may ultimately be subject to estate tax. Therefore, by simply employing the ILIT mechanism, you can avoid potentially losing about 50 percent of the proceeds to estate taxes.

In addition to a will (and a trust), I always recommend durable powers of attorney for you and your spouse. These documents name someone (the "attorney-in-fact") to make financial decisions for you, and survive your incapacity (this is the "durability" aspect). They can be written to be effective if you become incapacitated. However, this provision must be spelled out in the document; if not, the document will be effective immediately, and the named attorney-in-fact can then control all of your assets. So, typically, if a doctor is married for a long time, then I may suggest that the durable power of attorney be made effective immediately. If the parties have been married for a short period, or if the marriage is a second or third marriage, then the document will typically be made effective upon the doctor's disability (and the spouse may not be named as the attorney-in-fact).

Further, doctors and their spouses should sign advance medical directives, such as a designation of health care surrogate and a living will. In a declaration of health care surrogate, a person appoints an individual (typically the spouse) to make health care decisions for him or her if he or she is unable to do so. For example, if you need to give informed consent to an operation, but you are not in a position to do so, your spouse or someone else that you name can sign the informed consent for you.

In a living will, an individual can specify his or her intent as to desiring or avoiding life support if he or she is in a terminal condition, persistent vegetative state, or similar condition with no reasonable probability of recovery. Typically, in my practice, most clients choose to avoid life support in that situation. But some choose to be kept alive *under any circumstance. You can also choose a person to make the decision for you, based on your intent.*

Over your lifetime you will continually update these documents. So you need to make sure to fully understand them, review them from time to time, advise your attorney when life changes occur, and review them with your attorney every few years in any event.

Malpractice insurance is usually purchased with an agent that solely handles this professional liability insurance. In other words, this would be a different agent from the one that handles your life and disability insurance. Malpractice insurance should be purchased so that you are covered for any event that occurs while you covered by the insurance plan. This is called an occurrence policy. This means if you are sued fifteen years later for an event that happened during the coverage period, you are covered. You do not need to purchase a "tail" policy with this type of insurance. The other type of malpractice insurance is called "claims made" and only covers you while the policy is in effect. "Tail" insurance is necessary. It will protect you against claims that might occur afterwards but are related to the period of time the claims-made policy was in effect. When purchasing malpractice insurance, you should understand the limits. The policy will specify a per-claim coverage limit and also the aggregate limit for multiple claims within a set period of time. You should have a nice working relationship with your agent. It is not unusual to seek his or her guidance regarding a variety of malpractice issues that arise during your practice.

Corporate attorneys will help you with the many corporate issues that arise in your business. A health care attorney will help you avoid health-care-related legal issues. This is important, because medicine is a highly regulated industry. Problems such as stark law violations, HIPAA issues, physician reimbursement, and employment issues are examples of health-care-specific legal issues that will require a qualified health care attorney. Be certain that you hire a "board certified" health care attorney.

In summary, this chapter dealt with the first few critical steps of setting up your practice. These are decision-making steps that need to be started ten to twelve months before entering private practice. Critical points that were covered were: helping evaluate the opportunities between joining a solo practice or a group practice; understanding the different types of corporation structures; tips on how to trademark a corporate name; selecting a domain name; the importance of a line of credit; tips on hiring an accountant, lawyer, and insurance agent; and insurance options that should be evaluated. The next chapter will cover the regulatory aspects of your practice.

LICENSES, LAWS, AND ACRONYMS (DEA, NPI, CAQH, PECOS, HIPAA, HITECH, CLIA)

You are required by law to have a medical license before you start seeing patients. Some residency programs ensure that your license is active in the state that your residency program is in. However, if you are planning to move to a different state to set up practice, apply early for a license in that state. Residency programs may not remind you to do this before you graduate. You should. It will make a huge difference for you to have your license before you move there. If this is done early, it will help you with applying for hospital privileges, joining insurance plans, and evaluating job options.

Expect numerous delays and bureaucratic challenges when applying for your state medical license. Each state may have a different set of laws. You will have to contact each state's medical licensing board to determine its unique set of requirements and to request an application form. Be prepared to submit multiple documents, including your curriculum vitae (CV), proof of education, proof of licensure examination, prior employers, prior residences, and more. Your information must be accurate. Inaccuracies will slow down the licensing process.

Visit http://www.fsmb.org/fcvs.html to get the most up-to-date information regarding licensure in each state and requirements.

PEARL

Consider becoming a member of the Federation Credentials Verification Service (FCVS). If you ever change states, all of your information will be accessible and retrievable, stored in their database. The FCVS is a central database where organizations can obtain the record of the physician's credentials. The FCVS database allows you to create a lifetime professional record that can be modified and updated and forwarded at your request. Most but not all major licensing authorities accept documents for licensure verified by FCVS. FCVS can be contacted at 1-888-275-3287.

THE DRUG ENFORCEMENT AGENCY (DEA) LICENSE

PEARL

Even if you think you will not be prescribing controlled substances, apply early for a DEA number. Don't wait until you start practicing to apply for this license.

The DEA forms listed for registering can be found at:
http://www.deadiversion.usdoj.gov/drugreg/reg_apps/onlineforms.htm.
You will need to have the following information available in order to complete the form:
- Tax ID number and/or Social Security number;
- State controlled substance registration information;

- State medical license information;
- Credit card (VISA, MasterCard, Discover, or American Express)—the cost varies. It depends on the level and type of license you will be receiving.

THE NATIONAL PROVIDER IDENTIFIER NUMBER (NPI)

Apply for your NPI number (National Provider Identifier mumber) as soon as possible. The purpose of the NPI number is to uniquely identify you as a health care provider in standard transactions involving health care claims. These claims are the forms that you submit to insurance carriers to get paid for your patient services. Additionally, the NPI often is used on prescriptions, for coordination of benefits, in medical record systems, and in several other ways. You can't get paid without an NPI number. The Health Insurance Portability and Accountability Act (HIPAA) requires that any covered entity that transmits any electronic health information must have an NPI number.

The following information was retrieved from the CMS (Center for Medicare and Medicaid Services) Web site and provides the information you need to know to apply for an NPI number. It is free. A health care provider may apply for an NPI number in one of three ways:

Table 1. Process of applying for NPI (National Provider Identification) number

1. Apply through a Web-based application process. The Web address to the National Plan and Provider Enumeration System (NPPES) is https://nppes.cms.hhs.gov.

2. If requested, give permission to have an Electronic File Interchange Organization (EFIO) submit the application data on behalf of the health care provider (e.g., through

a bulk enumeration process). If a health care provider agrees to permit an EFIO to apply for the NPI, the EFIO will provide instructions regarding the information that is required to complete the process. More information on this option is available at: www.cms.hhs.gov.

3. Fill out and mail a paper application form to the NPI Enumerator. A copy of the application form (CMS-10114), which includes the NPI Enumerator's mailing address, is available only upon request through the NPI Enumerator. The NPI Enumerator's phone number is 1-800-465-3203 or TTY 1-800-692-2326.

When applying for an NPI, providers are encouraged to include their Medicare identifiers as well as those issued by any other health plans. If reporting a Medicaid identification number, include the associated state name. The legacy identifier information is critical for health plans in the development of crosswalks to aid in the transition to the NPI. Once the NPI application information has been submitted and the NPI assigned, NPPES (or an EFIO, if the health care provider was enumerated by way of an EFIO) will send the health care provider a notification that includes his or her NPI. This notification is proof of NPI enumeration and provides the information that will enable trading partners to verify a health care provider's NPI.

PITFALLS TO AVOID

Don't wait until you start seeing patients to apply for your NPI number; otherwise, you may not get paid.

THE COUNCIL FOR AFFORDABLE QUALITY HEALTHCARE (CAQH)

CAQH represents an initiative to simplify the process of health care administration and information exchange. It is meant to encourage administrative and clinical data integration. CAQH is a nonprofit alliance of health plans that offers an Online Application System (OAS) that is secure and free.

It is made available by the organizations and insurance companies that participate with CAQH initiatives.

Registering your personal information and completing your online application with CAQH will facilitate the process of applying to multiple health plans. It will avoid having to fill out multiple redundant forms with the same information on them. You can transmit your information electronically to CAQH participating health care plans (a number that is growing). Insurance companies that are not part of CAQH may be sent hard copies printed from the CAQH Web site.

THE PROVIDER ENROLLMENT, CHAIN, AND OWNERSHIP SYSTEM (PECOS).

The following information regarding PECOS was obtained from the CMS Web site:

The Centers for Medicare and Medicaid Services (CMS) has created a way for providers to enroll in Medicare online. The system for enrolling online is called the Internet-based Provider Enrollment, Chain, and Ownership System (PECOS). Internet-based PECOS is available to physicians, nonphysician practitioners, and provider and supplier organizations in all states and the District of Columbia. PECOS has a number of advantages over paper-based enrollment, and gives you quicker access to your enrollment information.

For physicians and nonphysician practitioners who already have an NPI, there are two basic steps to completing an enrollment action using Internet-based PECOS. Physicians and nonphysician practitioners must:

1. Go to Internet-based PECOS and complete, review, and submit the electronic enrollment application.
2. Print, sign, and date the two-page Certification Statement for each enrollment application you submit, and mail the Certification Statement and all supporting paper documentation to the Medicare contractor within seven days of electronic submission. Note: A Medicare contractor will not process an Internet enrollment application without the signed and dated Certification Statement. Signatures must be original and in ink (blue ink recommended). Copied or stamped signatures will not be accepted. In addition, the effective date of filing an enrollment application is the date your Medicare contractor receives the signed Certification Statement that is associated with the Internet submission.

For physicians and nonphysician practitioners who do not have an NPI, there are three basic steps to completing an enrollment action using Internet-based PECOS. Physicians and nonphysician practitioners must:

1. Have an NPPES User ID and password to use Internet-based PECOS. To create a Web user account and apply for an NPI at NPPES, go to https://nppes.cms.hhs.gov/NPPES/.
2. Once you have your NPI, go to Internet-based PECOS and complete, review, and submit the electronic enrollment application.

3. Print, sign, and date the 2-page Certification Statement for each enrollment application you submit, and mail the Certification Statement and all supporting paper documentation to the your Medicare contractor within 7 days of electronic submission. Note: A Medicare contractor will not process an Internet enrollment application without the signed and dated Certification Statement. Signatures must be original and in ink (blue ink recommended). Copied or stamped signatures will not be accepted. In addition, the effective date of filing an enrollment application is the date your Medicare contractor receives the signed Certification Statement that is associated with the Internet submission.

To be a registered user and log on to Internet-based PECOS, you must have the following:

- an active Web user account (user ID/password) established in the National Plan and Provider Enumeration System (NPPES);
- an active National Provider Identifier (NPI).

If you are a health care provider and do not have an NPI, apply for one at NPPES (https://nppes.cms.hhs.gov/).

If you do not have an active Web user account in NPPES, establish one by going to NPPES (https://nppes.cms.hhs.gov/).

If you need to update your account information, or if you have forgotten your user ID/password, please visit NPPES (https://nppes.cms.hhs.gov/).

If you are having issues with your user ID/password and are unable to log in, please contact the External User Services (EUS) Help Desk at 1-866-484-8049 or via e-mail at EUSSupport@cgi.com.

Physicians and nonphysician practitioners who wish to access Internet-based PECOS may go here: https://pecos.cms.hhs.gov

Please note that a hard copy Certification Statement (for security reasons) and all required documentation (license, DEA certificates, etc.) must still be mailed. This certification form and instructions will be on the PECOS Web site.

THE REGULATIONS

In this section, I will discuss the most relevant issues that impact your practice as they relate to new laws and regulations. I will not cover the laws in detail; rather, only as they apply to you managing your practice. I will cover the Health Insurance Portability and Accountability Act of 1996 (HIPAA), the new health care reform act called the American Recovery and Reinvestment Act of 2009 (ARRA 2009) , the Health Information Technology for Economic and Clinical Health (HITECH) Act's impact on HIPAA, and the Red Flags Rule.

HIPAA is a complex law. You are required to be in compliance. For the purpose of this book, I will not cover the entire law. However, I did select excerpts that are important and deserve highlighting. The following information was obtained from the Web site below and represents many of the most critical points for our purposes: http://www.hhs.gov/ocr/privacy/hipaa/understanding/summary/index.html.

The *Standards for Privacy of Individually Identifiable Health Information* ("Privacy Rule") establishes, for the first time, a set of national standards for the protection of certain health information. The U.S. Department of Health and Human Services ("HHS") issued the Privacy Rule to implement the requirement of the Health Insurance Portability and Accountability Act of 1996 ("HIPAA").

The Privacy Rule standards address the use and disclosure of an individual's health information—called "protected health information" by organizations subject to the Privacy Rule—called "covered entities," as well as standards for individuals' privacy rights to understand and control how their health information is used.

A major goal of the Privacy Rule is to assure that individuals' health information is properly protected while allowing the flow of health information needed to provide and promote high-quality health care and to protect the public's health and well-being. The rule strikes a balance that permits important uses of information, while protecting the privacy of people who seek care and healing.

Since, <u>as a doctor, you are considered a "covered entity,"</u> you are required by federal law to make sure your practice follows the rules of HIPAA and implements the required actions to be in compliance. If you are not in compliance, you will be subject to penalties and fines.

The following information was copied from the Department of Health and Human Services' OCR (Office of Civil Rights) Privacy Brief Summary of the HIPAA Privacy Rule:

PRINCIPLE FOR USES AND DISCLOSURES

Basic Principle. A major purpose of the Privacy Rule is to define and limit the circumstances in which an individual's protected heath information may be used or disclosed by covered entities. A covered entity may not use or disclose protected health information, except either: (1) as the Privacy Rule permits or requires; or (2) as the individual who is the subject of the information (or the individual's personal representative) authorizes in writing.

Required Disclosures. A covered entity must disclose protected health information in only two situations: (a) to individuals (or their personal representatives) specifically when they request access to, or an accounting of disclosures of, their protected health information; and (b) to HHS when it is undertaking a compliance investigation or review or enforcement action.

The HIPAA rule defines the term "business associate." As doctors, we have many "business associates." Business associates that might have access to our patients' information include our IT consultant, accountant, and various other services and vendors. We are required to have each business associate sign a "business associate agreement." This agreement states that the particular business associate will not share any of the personal health information he or she may see. This is a step you must do. Keep a copy of your business associate agreements accessible. HIPAA privacy rule defines a "business associate" as the following:

Business Associate Defined. In general, a business associate is a person or organization, other than a member of a covered entity's workforce, that performs certain functions or activities on behalf of, or provides certain services to, a covered entity that involve the use or disclosure of individually identifiable health information. Business associate functions or activities on behalf of a covered entity include claims processing, data analysis, utilization review, and billing. Business associate services to a covered entity are limited to legal, actuarial, accounting, consulting, data aggregation, management, administrative, accreditation, or financial services. However, persons or organizations are not considered business associates if their functions or services do not involve the use or disclosure of protected health information, and where any access to protected health information by such persons would be incidental, if at all. A covered entity can be the business associate of another covered entity.

Also, the rule requires the following, according to the Department of Health and Human Services' OCR Privacy Summary:

> **Business Associate Contract.** When a covered entity uses a contractor or other nonworkforce member to perform *'business associate'* services or activities, the Rule requires that the covered entity include certain protections for the information in a business associate agreement (in certain circumstances governmental entities may use alternative means to achieve the same protections). In the business associate contract, a covered entity must impose specified written safeguards on the individually identifiable health information used or disclosed by its business associates. Moreover, a covered entity may not contractually authorize its business associate to make any use or disclosure of protected health information that would violate the Rule. Covered entities that have an existing written contract or agreement with business associates prior to October 15, 2002, which is not renewed or modified prior to April 14, 2003, are permitted to continue to operate under that contract until they renew the contract or April 14, 2004, whichever is first. A sample business associate contract language is available on the OCR website at: http://www.hhs.gov/ocr/hipaa/contractprov.html. Also see OCR 'Business Associate' Guidance.

The following are the permitted uses of an individual's personal health information by a covered entity as described in the OCR privacy summary:

Permitted Uses and Disclosures. A covered entity is permitted, but not required, to use and disclose protected health information, without an individual's authorization, for the following purposes or situations: (1) To the Individual (unless required for access or accounting of disclosures); (2) Treatment, Payment, and Health Care Operations; (3) Opportunity to Agree or Object; (4) Incident to an otherwise permitted use and disclosure; (5) Public Interest and Benefit Activities; and (6) Limited Data Set for the purposes of research, public health, or health care operations. Covered entities may rely on professional ethics and best judgments in deciding which of these permissive uses and disclosures to make.

The Department of Health and Human Services' OCR Privacy Summary states that you must provide the following as it relates to HIPAA:

1. **Privacy Practices Notice**. Each covered entity, with certain exceptions, must provide a notice of its privacy practices.

2. **Acknowledgment of Notice Receipt.** A covered health care provider with a direct treatment relationship with individuals must make a good-faith effort to obtain written acknowledgment from patients of receipt of the privacy practices notice.

3. **Business Associate Contract.** When a covered entity uses a contractor or other nonworkforce member to perform *"business associate"* services or activities, the Rule requires that the covered entity include certain protections for the information in a business associate agreement (in certain circumstances governmental

entities may use alternative means to achieve the same protections).

4. **Privacy Policies and Procedures.** A covered entity must develop and implement written privacy policies and procedures that are consistent with the Privacy Rule.

5. **Privacy Personnel.** A covered entity must designate a privacy official responsible for developing and implementing its privacy policies and procedures, and a contact person or contact office responsible for receiving complaints and providing individuals with information on the covered entity's privacy practices.

6. **Authorization.** A covered entity must obtain the individual's written authorization for any use or disclosure of protected health information that is not for treatment, payment or health care operations or otherwise permitted or required by the Privacy Rule.

7. **Workforce Training and Management.** Workforce members include employees, volunteers, trainees, and may also include other persons whose conduct is under the direct control of the entity (whether or not they are paid by the entity). A covered entity must train all workforce members on its privacy policies and procedures, as necessary and appropriate for them to carry out their functions.

The American Recovery and Reinvestment Act of 2009 (ARRA 2009) embodied President's Obama's mission of changing health care. However, it is a very complex and detailed law that impacts practitioners from many different angles. I will attempt to provide you with the "nuts and bolts" of the law. You should understand how it impacts your practice of medicine and your patients. In the following section, I am not rendering an opinion on this law or the current political rhetoric. Time will be the best judge.

How does the law affect doctors?

Although I never believe that any politician will actually increase physician payments, supposedly Medicare will give extra payments to physicians and nurses providing care in areas with doctor shortages. This will benefit doctors in forty-two states. Somehow, paperwork requirements are to be simplified to enable doctors to have more time with their patients. Student loans will be "forgiven" for those medical students that provide primary care in needed areas. Medicare physicians may be paid according to "quality" and not "quantity" of services provided.

Where do the savings come from?

Section 3601 of the new law states that nothing in the new law can cut current Medicare benefits. The law provides for an "independent" Medicare advisory board that is projected to save the program $16 billion over ten years. Additionally, by cracking down on fraud and waste, an additional $7 billion is to be saved. Innovations, electronic health records, and bonus payments are all felt to contribute to long-term savings.

According to an excellent article by Patricia Barry in the AARP bulletin, the most important things you need to know about the new law are that it: helps 32 million Americans get insurance; makes insurance companies not deny coverage for preexisting medical conditions; guarantees basic benefits for everyone in Medicare, such as preventive free services and reducing the "doughnut hole" in the part D drug program; "leaves medical decisions" in the hands of you and your doctor; requires most people to have health insurance coverage by 2014; creates state-run insurance exchanges for people that are uninsured, self-employed, or between jobs; offers immediate tax credits to small businesses; and keeps Medicare financially sound for ten more years while reducing the deficit by $143 billion.

She points out five things that may be surprising to you in the law: members of Congress will be required to buy health plans through state-run exchanges as of 2014, illegal immigrants are prohibited from buying health insurance through exchanges, chain restaurants and vending machines must post calorie counts for their foods, tanning parlor services will have a 10 percent sales tax, and new long-term care insurance will let you make contributions for future cash benefits for help to remain in your home.

If your patient is currently enrolled in Medicare, then the new law guarantees that existing benefits will not change. Starting in 2011, traditional Medicare enrollees will receive annual physicals and preventive services for free. Patients will receive $250 toward the coverage gap for drug costs. In 2011, patients will receive a 50 percent discount on brand name and biologic drugs when purchased while in the gap. People with higher incomes will be required to pay higher premiums for drug coverage. There will be no change in Medigap supplemental insurance.

If your patient receives employer insurance, then he or she may keep his or her current plan. He or she will not be forced into a "government" plan. Starting this year (2010), insurance companies can no longer place lifetime caps on your care. Also, insurance companies will have to spend 85 percent of premiums on medical care, not profits or overhead. Starting in 2013, wellness incentives may be offered to create employee discounts. Also, the maximum allowed to be contributed to flexible spending accounts will be $2,500 per year. Accounts may no longer be used to buy over-the-counter medicines that are not prescribed by a physician.

If your patient is uninsured, then the patient may be able to buy coverage through an immediate but temporary high-risk program. Insurers can no longer drop coverage if premiums have been paid. Children may not be denied coverage due to preexisting conditions. Starting in 2014, insurers can charge older patients no more than three times the amount they charge younger adults. Patients will be able to select from a menu of choices offered through an insurance exchange run by the state.

The Health Information Technology for Economic and Clinical Health (HITECH) Act became law when the American Recovery and Revinvestment Act of 2009 was passed by Congress. HITECH affects the way your office deals with HIPAA compliance and holds physicians to more stringent requirements as they relate to data breach rule requirements. HITECH mandates how practices must maintain and protect personal health information (PHI). Specifically, it requires documentation, such as logs of qualifying breaches in PHI. Breaches might include accidental disclosure, intentional disclosures, or theft of PHI data. After a qualifying breach has occurred, a practice must prove that is has made all required notifications. In general, the notice must be in plain language and include: date of the breach and discovery, brief description of what happened, brief description of information involved, steps the affected individuals should take to protect themselves, a brief description of the practice's remedial actions, and, lastly, the contact information for affected individuals to gain more information. As a result of HITECH, more severe penalties will be enforced for HIPAA violations. The details of HITECH are beyond the scope of this book. A policy for your practice should be established and reviewed with an attorney.

STAT CONSULT FROM JEFF COHEN, BOARD-CERTIFIED HEALTH CARE ATTORNEY

Information technology (IT) and electronic medical records (EMR) are at the core of health care reform. The thinking is that technology will (1) ensure communication between providers, (2) allow providers to measure and control costs, and (3) enable providers to measure and control quality and outcomes.

The so-called "HITECH" provisions of the federal health care reform law create a pot of about $34 billion worth of incentive payments for eligible professionals and hospitals that attain meaningful use of certified electronic health care records (EHR) technology. To obtain any money, eligible parties will have to demonstrate full compliance no later than 2015, and earlier (2011!) if they want the full benefit. Medicare has allocated roughly $44,000 worth of incentives for each compliant physician, and Medicaid offers another $20,000, roughly, but the real incentive is not the incentive money; it's the fact that financial penalties apply if you don't comply by 2015.

Financial incentives are available for eligible professionals who use certified HIT which satisfies the "meaningful use" regulations, which were issued August 2010. They are complex and limited by time lines which industry insiders claim to be unreachable.

The long-awaited "meaningful use" regulations are an important step in the process of weaving health information technology into the fabric of U.S. health care policy and delivery. The regs take into account over two thousand comments and begin the process of actually using electronic records in health care settings.

According to the new regs, eligible providers (including physicians) are subject to twenty-five specific criteria, while hospitals are subject to twenty-three. The final rule sets forth standard formats for clinical summaries and prescriptions; defines terms to describe clinical problems, procedures and lab tests, medications, and allergies; and establishes security safeguards for exchange of electronic health information over the Internet. In general, the final rule is designed to give professionals and hospitals greater flexibility in demonstrating meaningful use of certified EHR technology. The flexibility arises out of the rule's three-step process. The final rule establishes Stage One. A Stage Two update is scheduled for the end of 2011. A Stage Three update is set for the end of 2013.

At this time, eligible professionals must meet a core group of fifteen required objectives, including:

1. use of computerized provider entry for at least 30 percent of all unique patients with at least one medication in their medication list seen by their physician;

2. implementation of drug-drug and drug-allergy interaction checks;

3. recording and charting changes in vitals, blood pressure, and body mass index for at least 50 percent of all unique patients between two and twenty;

4. recording smoking status of 50 percent of all patients over thirteen; and

5. provision of clinical summaries to patients of each office visit within three business days of the visit for at least 50 percent of all office visits.

Two certifying bodies have now been approved: CCHIT (from Chicago, Illinois) and Drummond Group (Austin, Texas). The certifying bodies will certify whether a specific IT solution satisfies the "meaningful use" regs, which will surely continue to evolve. As such, physicians should use caution, since vendors are selling and physicians are buying software and solutions in hopes they will qualify for the incentive payments. Physicians should make sure that their contracts with such vendors protect them by requiring the solutions to be certified and meet the meaningful use guidelines. Moreover, their contracts with the IT vendors should contain provisions like:

1. *the IT solution is certified by CCHIT or Drummond;*

2. *the vendor will ensure continuous compliance;*

3. *the solution will qualify the user for incentive payments; and*

4. *the vendor will stand behind those promises with the pertinent indemnification provisions.*

Every physician office should have a security protocol. This should include a written computer and network security manual. The manual must have listed in it your policies for catastrophic data recovery. Catastrophic recovery means the process by which you will restore patient data in the event it is lost. You must have written policies and procedures for maintaining privacy and security. You should have access privileges to data and software defined by position. You will need to list who is the main administrator and who has which passwords. Your manual should describe how you are protecting your data and your network from viruses and hackers.

Table 2. Contents of Computer, Network, and Security Manual

1. Privacy policies

2. Security policies

3. Password policies

4. Administrative policies

5. E-mail policies for employees

6. Computer access policies

7. User privilege policies for each position

8. Redundancy protocols

9. Emergency backup and restore policies

10. Antiviral precautions and policies

11. Precautions to prevent hacking or unintended disclosures

12. Network topography

13. Listing of all hardware

14. Listing of software licenses

15. Maintenance and update schedules

In general, your network and computer security policy should address the following areas on a regular basis: evaluating security measures and improving and updating when necessary; strengthening password protection; reviewing your practice performance to ensure all safeguards are followed; securing areas where data are located; installing and maintaining firewalls; and backing up your data regularly.

Physicians are not yet but may be required to be compliant with the Red Flags Rule. There is discussion between the AMA (American Medical Association) and the Federal Trade Commission (FTC) to clarify the Red Flags Rule as it applies to physician offices. It is the AMA's assertion that physician offices are not creditors. I am including this section since, at the time of this writing, doctors may still be required to be compliant in 2010.

The following information was summarized from the practice management section of the AMA's Web site. This document was prepared by the AMA to help physicians understand the Red Flags Rule.

The purpose of the Red Flags Rule is to require certain entities to develop and implement policies and procedures to protect against identity theft. The Red Flags Rule applies to any creditor, and since the Federal Trade Commission (FTC) considers physicians who accept insurance or allow payment plans to be creditors. The FTC then subjects physicians to the Red Flags Rule.

The Red Flags Rule and HIPAA are different, though they share some things in common. HIPAA is intended to protect personal health information (PHI) for security and privacy purposes. PHI is defined by HIPAA and is covered by the Red Flags Rule, but the rule extends to other sensitive information that HIPAA doesn't cover, such as: credit card information; tax identification numbers, Social Security numbers, business identification numbers, and employer identification numbers; insurance claim information; and background checks for employees and service providers.

A red flag is a pattern, practice, or specific account activity that indicates the possibility of identity theft. The FTC identifies the following as red flags: alerts, notifications, or warnings from a consumer reporting agency; suspicious documents and/or personal identifying information, such as an inconsistent address or nonexistent Social Security number; unusual use of, or suspicious activity relating to, a patient account; notices of possible identity theft from patients, victims of identity theft, or law enforcement authorities.

Table 3. Procedures for identifying and responding to red flags:

1. Identify what red flags can occur in your practice.

2. Identify how you will detect red flags.

3. Establish a procedure for responding to red flags.

4. Review and update your practice's red flags policy and manual annually.

5. Incorporate specific administrative elements into your red flags program.

THE OFFICE LOGS

This is the only section in the book that deals with the "practice" of medicine versus the "business" of medicine. I suggest that you set QA (Quality Assurance) and QC (Quality Control) logs before you see your first patient. If you take the time initially to set up a "checks and balances" system for your practice, then you are less likely to make a mistake later. Although different specialties will have different needs, in general, logs, either in paper or electronic form, will be invaluable to your practice. Start the first day. Make it a daily habit to review and maintain these logs.

Depending upon your specialty, you may need a log to track and monitor lab and biopsy results. These are referred to as QC (Quality Control) logs. The log should reflect when and who reviewed the lab result. It should also record the action taken. The log records the date and time a specimen was taken and when the result was given. If you create this log, then you are less likely to miss an abnormal result. It might seem trivial at first, but as your practice grows, you may have hundreds of results that need to be addressed every week. They should be addressed routinely. It is critical that this process is established as protocol to avoid a reporting error.

I would also suggest a separate log for monitoring medications for side effects. This log would include any interventions that the medication requires. Some medications require monthly liver function tests, for example. If this is the case, your log should help you monitor this so you do not overlook it.

Quality assurance (QA) logs help ensure that your lab's testing procedures and equipment are reviewed regularly for quality and reliability. This requirement includes proficiency testing results of required personnel, such as lab directors, lab managers, lab technicians, and clinicians. Proficiency testing is the demonstration that specific personnel are being checked for their proficiency to perform a specific lab function or test. QA and QC logs are part of your CLIA (Clinical Laboratory Improvement Amendment) obligations.

Additional logs include establishing a Medicare or billing compliance program. Compliance programs are only valuable if you follow them. The compliance program should require the appointment of a compliance officer. The program should help employees and patients file complaints with the practice if improper billing activities are suggested. It should include regular training of staff regarding proper coding, chart documentation, avoidance of fraudulent activities, and general billing matters. The compliance program should be set up initially with your other practice logs. It should be reviewed regularly and periodically.

In summary, this chapter reviewed the impact of the new health care regulations on your practice of medicine. In particular, we covered HIPAA, the HITECH act, ARRA 2009, and the Red Flags Rule. We discussed preparations you need to take to be in compliance with these rules. We also covered security protocols and precautions that you should take as they relate to implementing technology. Lastly, we touched upon the importance of maintaining logs for the practice of medicine and CLIA. In the next chapter, we will discuss the nuances of obtaining managed care opportunities and hospital privileges.

HOSPITAL PRIVILEGES, MEDICARE, AND MANAGED CARE PLANS

PEARL

Do not wait until you move to your new location to apply for hospital privileges.

Here are a few reasons to start the process early of applying for hospital privileges.

1. Many insurance plans require hospital privileges to verify your credentials and expertise.
2. Hospitals are the best place to network with administration, nurses, and other doctors. The earlier they get to know you, the sooner they may refer patients to you.
3. If you start seeing patients and you need to send them to the hospital, it is important to have privileges so that you can admit patients to the hospital.

This process can be slow and political. You may find that local doctors may be threatened by you and try to block your privileges and application. You need to be persistent.

PEARL

Befriend the director of physician staff services for the hospital. This person will be invaluable. He or she can help you navigate through the application process and an understanding of the politics of the hospital. He or she can be an invaluable ally for you.

STAT CONSULT FROM JEFF COHEN, BOARD-CERTIFIED HEALTH CARE ATTORNEY

Medical Staff Issues

Physicians have to be well informed about their relationship with hospitals where they are on staff. Doctors whose practices bring them into contact with hospitals sometimes feel they are living "in the mouth of the lion." Still, the nature of their practices requires close and cooperative working relationships. For most, this means some give and take, but they work. For a few, it means all-out war, which is exactly what one doctor found in Naples. Lucky for him, he knew his legal rights well enough to fight the hospital…and to win.

The Naples doctor was a neurologist and a pain management specialist who practiced at the hospital without a contract. An anesthesia group obtained an exclusive contract at the hospital to provide anesthesia and pain management services. When the doctor's two-year grant of privileges was up and he reapplied for the same privileges he had held, the hospital denied him (without a hearing) the right to continue practicing at the hospital.

The doctor sued the hospital to allow him to continue practicing at the hospital. He argued, among other things, that the hospital owed him a hearing before his privileges could be taken. Though the trial court agreed and granted him the right to a hearing, the hospital appealed the ruling. On appeal, the Florida court found that in fact the medical staff rules and regulations did not give the doctor the right to a hearing. Fortunately, however, the appellate court decided that a hearing would be meaningless and that the hospital had no legitimate grounds to deny his reapplication for pain management privileges.

The case is extremely important for a couple of reasons. First, it reaffirms the long-held view in Florida that medical staff bylaws and rules and regulations are a contract between a hospital and a medical staff. Second, it underscores the importance of how those documents are worded. For instance, the doctor did not have a right to a hearing when his reapplication was denied. Unlike many medical staffs, the language simply was not contained in the bylaws, rules, and regulations.

The case is yet another wake-up call for physicians and hospitals alike. Medical staff privileges in Florida are sacred and cannot be impaired in any way unless (1) the medical staff bylaws, rules, and regulations are strictly followed, or (2) the doctor has entered into a contract with the hospital that allows the hospital to terminate his or her medical staff privileges on terms other than what is described in the medical staff bylaws, rules, and regulations. Both medical staffs and hospitals should carefully review their bylaws, rules, and regulations. They have to be very clear about termination provisions when exclusive agreements are entered into.

The hospital should represent and warrant that it has the ability to enter into an exclusive agreement. And, finally, every doctor must remember that, unless he or she has a contract with a hospital that allows it, he or she cannot be forced off a medical staff without a fair hearing.

Other key areas for medical staffs to consider pertain to (1) peer review activity and (2) conflicts of interest within medical staff leadership. Being investigated by the peer review committee of a hospital is one of the most stressful things a physician can experience. Yet, knowing a little law and exercising some common sense can help dramatically.

Peer review activity is authorized by both federal and state law. The reason for the laws is to ensure that patients are well cared for in licensed health care facilities. As such, the laws make peer review fairly simple for the reviewing facility. For instance, facilities must provide the affected physician written notice and afford the physician a "fair hearing" with certain procedural benefits, such as the right to examine and cross-examine witnesses, and also the right to submit a written statement upon the close of the hearing.

The laws cloak the process in confidentiality in hopes that this will encourage participants to be honest and feel free to actively participate in the process. And if the facilities provide the affected physician a fair hearing by following the procedural requirements of the laws, the facilities and those who testify in the process are immune from liability for antitrust violations. Peer review is intended to resolve quality concerns on an intra-professional basis. Moreover, it is easy for the health care facility to comply with the applicable laws. Finally, lawsuits against health *care facilities in connection with peer review have rarely, if ever, been successful. From the affected physician's perspective, the reviewing facility has a huge advantage.*

In truth, practically speaking, peer review is a last resort. It arises typically after multiple committees have reviewed the concern and usually after many discussions with the affected physician. A matter goes to peer review usually out of the medical staff's perception that its quality concerns are not being heard or taken seriously by the affected physician.

Nevertheless, affected physicians have a great deal of control in the matter, and the outcome will depend largely on how they view the process and participate in it. For instance, if the doctor views the process as a personal attack, it will be difficult to participate meaningfully and positively. The trick for the affected physician is to not take the process personally. If the physician takes the position of "You're wrong; and I'll fight you," the process will be adversarial and the outcome will be painful. If, instead, the affected doctor takes the position of "Help me to understand and address your concerns," the process can be smooth and the outcome can be positive, even beneficial. This is not to say that affected physicians should simply lie down. In fact, that will be as unhelpful as being combative. Instead, seek to understand and communicate.

Many physicians are motivated in the peer review process by fear associated with a report to the National Practitioner Data Bank (NPDB). NPDB reporting is basically triggered by peer review activity that involves quality issues. If, however, the doctor allows the fear of an NPDB report to control him or her, it will typically lead to the physician hardening his position in the process. In other words, the fear of an NPDB report often causes a physician to lose his or her best advantages: an open mind and willingness to discuss and compromise. In truth, an NPDB report is not a death knell to a physician's professional career. In fact, the doctor has the right to respond to an NPDB report, and the response will be available to those who query the NPDB. Affected physicians should remember that nearly every doctor who has been sued or who settles a claim has been reported to the NPDB, no matter how ludicrous the claim may be. Still, NPDB reports can raise questions and are upsetting. As such, affected doctors should address the medical staff's concerns at the earliest opportunity. In fact, the best way to avoid NPDB reporting is to simply address the medical staff's concerns before the matter rises to the level of peer review.

With the foregoing in mind, affected physicians should keep the following tips in mind:

> *Take committee action and quality concerns seriously before they rise to the level of the MEC or peer review committee.*

> *Seek to understand quality concerns rather than take them personally or attack. The approach for successful litigation does not usually work in peer review matters.*

> *Seek opportunities to meet with the medical staff and address its concerns, even once peer review activity is under way.*

As far as conflicts of interest (COI) go, medical staffs are increasingly frustrated with the financial relationships their medical executive committee (MEC) members have with the hospitals where they work. These financial relationships can be the cause of troubling conflicts of interest. Medical staffs need to be proactive about the issue.

A hospital based physician's livelihood (and the economic welfare of his or her family) depends in part on having a good relationship with the administration of the hospital where he or she works. It is easy, therefore, to see how the physician would be hard pressed to go against the hospital on controversial matters. The same goes for a full-time employed physician of a hospital and even a medical director who may derive significant compensation from his or her relationship with the hospital.

Looked at another way, what about a physician who staffs a hospital-based department at hospital #1 who wants to get on staff of competing hospital #2? What about the physician who is employed by hospital #1 becoming a member of hospital #2 and who wants to become president of hospital 2's medical staff?

Intertwined financial relationships between hospitals and physician are on the rise. The complexity of an ever-evolving business model brings hospitals and physicians closer and closer, which creates significant COIs. MECs must take a good look at what circumstances constitute a COI and develop methods to counteract them.

A COI basically exists for an MEC member when the member has a relationship with a party which causes the member to place his or her personal interests before those interests of the medical staff as a whole. A classic COI is a financial relationship with the hospital. If an MEC member receives money from a hospital for providing a service to or on behalf of a hospital, a COI exists. But the inquiry does not stop there. Simply having a COI is not dispositive. The question is what to do about it.

There is essentially a two-step process involved for an MEC member with a COI. First, the COI must be disclosed. This ought to be done annually and at each MEC meeting. Second, on any matter where the COI is implicated, the MEC member ought to recuse himself or herself from a vote on the matter. He or she can participate in the MEC consideration, but should leave the room when the vote is taken.

There is a third option, a poison pill of sorts. If an MEC member finds that the COI has him or her bouncing in and out of the MEC meeting room regularly, there ought to be consideration given to the person's resignation.

At the very least, medical staffs must develop policies and procedures regarding COIs. They ought to be defined and handled on a predetermined basis. Moreover, medical staffs should give serious consideration to ensuring that at least a majority of the MEC members do not have a COI that would prevent them from doing their job, which is to ensure the integrity and proper functioning of the medical staff.

MEDICARE

You have three options as a provider dealing with Medicare.

The first option is that you can choose to be a participating provider. A participating provider receives payments directly from CMS (Center for Medicare and Medicaid Services). This is called accepting assignments, and you must follow the billing rules to get paid for your services. Participating providers must accept Medicare's allowed charge as payment in full. Medicare covers 80 percent of a patient's allowed amount, and the patient is responsible for the remaining 20 percent. This may be covered by a secondary insurer or by the patient entirely. Most practicing physicians accept assignment and are participating providers.

The second option is nonparticipating status. This status permits you to charge your patients additional fees up to the Medicare limiting charge. Patients covered by Medicare will receive a check directly from Medicare. You must collect payment directly from the patient. In this option, providers may accept assignment on a case-by-case basis. If CMS pays a nonparticipating provider directly, it will reduce the amount paid by 5 percent. This is because Medicare-approved amounts for services provided by nonparticipating providers are set at 95 percent of Medicare-approved amounts for participating providers. Nonparticipating providers may charge more than the approved amount but are limited to 115 percent of Medicare-approved amounts. By the time bad debts, collection costs, and claim processing are calculated, the differences become much less significant.

I choose to be a participating provider for many reasons. Some of the procedures I perform are too expensive for patients to pay the difference in price. I would have to negotiate that difference away. Additionally, payment is faster from Medicare and secondary insurers. And, directories of participating physicians are provided to senior citizen groups and individuals, making it easier for them to find you as a doctor.

Physicians that may wish to change their status from participating to nonparticipating may do so annually.

THE MANAGED CARE PLAN

It can take several months to be approved as a provider for a particular managed care plan. Start this process early. You will need to learn which plans pay best in your location. A good place to learn this is by speaking to other doctors in the area. Ask them what plans they accept and how well they pay. This is important if you are a specialist. You rely on physician referrals for patients. Doctors do not want to send patients to a specialist who will not accept their patient's insurance. You should participate in the same managed care plans as your referring doctors.

After you have discovered which plans your potential referring doctors participate in, contact the plans. There will be process for you to follow to become a participating provider. Do your research carefully. If you join the wrong plan or make the wrong deal with a managed care company, it can have disastrous consequences for your practice.

When I first started my practice, I joined as many managed care plans as I could. I was scared that if I didn't participate in managed care, then I would have no patients. However, that fear was unfounded. As my practice grew, my reliance on the managed care plans for patients dwindled. I was fortunate because of the location and demographics of my practice. I lived and practiced in an area with a high concentration of retirees and elderly. As a result, most of my patients were Medicare insured. I was able to "wean" off of the managed care plans early. Most physicians, either due to their specialty type or their practice location, will not be able to avoid participating with managed care plans. If you are one of these physicians and you cannot avoid managed care, then you need to understand the realities of managed care reimbursement. I learned this the hard way.

The first few years of my practice I participated in managed care plan "XYZ." This plan contracted to pay me 80 percent of the Medicare allowable fee schedule. Each month I had to fight to get reimbursement from plan "XYZ." A common tactic of managed care plans is to reject or delay paying your claims for reasons that are unclear. The office biller or the billing service is forced to resubmit the claim or fight the rejection. This process caused payments to be delayed from weeks to several months. It does not matter if you are billing internally or using a billing service. In both scenarios, the collection of these fees becomes more and more difficult due to the delays. It is easy to overlook your collections from one particular insurer. The amount grows because you continue to see patients from those plans. You believe that you are getting 80 percent of Medicare allowable. You may think the plan is great because you are getting a constant flow of patients. However, after careful analysis, you will see that because of delays in payments, denials of claims, resubmission of claims, and work related to fighting the insurance denials, your compensation from the plans turns out to be much less than the original agreed amount. You must be prepared to fight for every penny. I was not. I was too busy seeing other patients to fight for the money I was owed. We did send a few letters from an attorney threatening action. The insurance companies are prepared. They know that most doctors do not have the time or money to fight them. The amounts due are not high enough to justify the effort for both the lawyers and the doctors. The managed care plans understand this and have the advantage.

After a few years and a loss of approximately $30,000, I decided to terminate the relationship with the managed care plan. This was the scariest and yet the best move I made. It was scary to terminate a relationship with an insurance plan that accounted for 25 percent of patients in the practice. I did not know if I would be able to sustain that loss of patient volume. Additionally, I thought I might lose referrals from doctors for their Medicare (and nonmanaged care) patients. I no longer accepted "XYZ" patients' insurance. My worries turned out to be false. This may not be the case for other doctors. Most other specialties are more dependent on managed care than I was.

I suggest contracting with "fee for service" managed care plans. These are plans that pay you a discounted fixed rate off the Medicare allowable fee schedule. The Medicare fee schedule varies by geography. It is the standard upon which most insurance plans base their fee schedules. In the early days of managed care, reimbursement was higher than the Medicare allowable. However, times have changed. Occasionally, if you are fortunate and your specialty is in need or in short supply in your community, you will have more "negotiating" power. You may be able to negotiate a more favorable rate.

The other type of managed care plan is the "at risk" or "capitated" plan. In this sort of plan, an insurance provider will pay you a set fee per month to see a set number of patients. So, if there are ten thousand patients on the plan in your community, you agree to be available to see all or a part of that number. This is called an "at risk" plan because you are getting a set payment without knowing how many patient visits you will have. In a month that you see fewer patients, you make more money per patient visit. The converse is true if you see more patients that month. The danger with this type of arrangement is that the patient load can overwhelm your practice. It can take up all your time. This may keep you from seeing patients with more attractive payment plans.

There are pitfalls that need to be avoided when signing a provider agreement with an insurance company. I suggest you review your first few contracts with a health care attorney. Be certain you do not sign an agreement with clauses that can come back and haunt you.

PEARL

Before you sign a provider agreement, make sure you do the following:

1. Read the "hold harmless" clause carefully. Most malpractice carriers make you remove the "hold harmless" clause from the insurance plans so that you do not hold the insurance plan harmless. If you do not remove this clause and your malpractice carrier has exclusion for this, then you may be putting yourself at risk.

2. Read the "termination" clause so that you understand how much notice you must give to the insurance plan upon termination. There are several legal issues to be careful of here. If you decide to terminate because you are not getting paid according to your agreement, you need to make sure

that you don't "abandon" (a legal term) your patients. Therefore, you must go through a notification process and understand it before terminating. Typically, you have to give patients thirty to sixty days to find another provider. You must provide care for thirty to sixty days after you have given notice of termination. Obviously, you want to make this period of time as short as possible without "abandoning" patient care responsibilities. You might have to fight to get paid by the insurance plan during this termination period.

3. Read the insurance company's termination options. What gives it the right to terminate you? For example, if you decide to leave a hospital and change to a different one, does that create a termination event with the insurance company?

4. Never sign any part of this agreement personally. Always make sure your signature is representative of the corporation and practice name.

5. Review and understand what the company's policies are for "disputes" under payment.

6. Make sure that the contract contains nothing that compromises your principles or mandates how to care for patients with certain problems.

7. Review what your call, cross-coverage, and vacation responsibilities are.

8. Ask for and review a sample of the company's payment schedule and fees paid to doctors based on commonly used codes. Confirm that the amounts are what you expect.

9. Review what their policies are if you have a physician assistant or nurse practitioner seeing the company's covered patients.

10. Find out if you are required to send to a specific lab. Ask yourself if that lab meets your criteria for quality.

11. Review the company's policies on patient records and ensure you have all the rights to retain patient records once the contract has been terminated.

12. Make sure that you have the right to terminate your relationship with the patient at any time. Review the period of time after you terminate the contract that you are obligated to continue to see the patient.

13. Make sure nothing in the contract prohibits the patient from seeing you after you terminate the contract.

STAT CONSULT FROM JEFF COHEN, BOARD-CERTIFIED HEALTHCCARE ATTORNEY

Managed Care Contracting

Managed care contracts are an entirely different matter with their own pitfalls. Managed care contracts usually suffer from two common problems: (1) very important terms are unclear, and (2) the cost control provisions are unfair. In contracting with payers, as in any contract, specificity matters. If the contract is not crystal clear on an issue, the parties can expect to fight about it, sometimes in expensive litigation. Similarly, ensuring fairness in a contract can prevent disputes.

Clarity

Definitions. This is usually the first part of a contract, and it may seem innocuous enough, but certain definitions are key to physicians. In particular, definitions of covered services, emergency services, members, and participating providers usually need work.

The definition of covered services should specify the services to be provided by the physician. Otherwise, the physician could be financially responsible for services he or she does not provide. For instance, does the term include diagnostic services or therapy? If not, be clear that such services are not covered. One way to be clear about the matter is to specify the CPT codes.

Emergency services should be linked to the judgment of a layperson rather than the hindsight of the payer. That is, a layperson is the one who decides to rush to a physician's office or a hospital emergency department. Since federal law requires hospitals and their medical staffs to screen and stabilize any emergency medical condition, there is no choice involved in treating someone who may have a serious problem. Moreover, since the expenditure of resources is necessary to see if there is an emergency medical condition in the first place, the fact that one did not really exist after all does not resolve the issue of the resources and time spent find that out. As such, one definition to consider inserting in place of the usual contractual language is:

" 'Emergency medical condition' means a condition manifesting itself by symptoms of sufficient severity such that the absence of immediate medical attention, in the judgment of a reasonably prudent lay person prior to an initial medical screening and in the judgment of a reasonably prudent physician after the screening, could be expected to result in serious impairment or dysfunction of any bodily function, organ, or part."

The definition of what constitutes a member is also tricky. In particular, physicians should be wary of getting stuck providing services to people who they reasonably believed were members of a payer, but who turned out not to be. One approach is to require the payer to give members identification cards and periodically updated lists of members. For instance, the following type of provision might be helpful:

"Notwithstanding the foregoing and any provision of this Agreement to the contrary, however, all such Members shall present an appropriate identification card and/or identify the appropriate preferred network/payer at the time of preauthorization. Otherwise, no discount as set forth in this Agreement shall apply; and [Participating Provider] shall be entitled to bill and collect its full charges. [Payer/Plan] agrees to provide [Participating Provider] timely and accurate lists of Participating Providers and Members.

Similarly, the definition of a participating provider is key, since failing to refer to a physician who is contracted with the patient's plan can result in financial penalties to the referring physician. As such, the same types of obligations mentioned above regarding members should be created concerning participating providers. That is, the plan should give you periodically updated lists of physicians who participate.

Fairness

In addition to the need for clarity, most managed care agreements lack what many consider to be basic procedural fairness. For instance, most agreements contain provisions that permit the plan to implement any rules, regulations, policies, and procedures the plan desires at any time. The physician does not necessarily know about these things, and such things can undermine the very language of the contract. To meet these concerns, the following should be helpful:

"[Participating Provider's] agreement to be bound by such [policies, procedures, rules, or regulations] shall be contingent upon [Participating Provider] being provided advanced written notice of any proposed adverse decision or event and a reasonable opportunity to respond to such proposal. Moreover, the parties agree that to the extent the foregoing conflicts with the terms of this Agreement, the terms of this Agreement shall govern."

Physician complaints regarding payer payment practices are constantly heard, and there are some provisions to consider in preventing those problems, such as:

"Notwithstanding any provision of this Agreement to the contrary, Payer agrees to ensure that all clean claims are paid within thirty days. 'Clean Claims' are those which meet the HCFA requirements. If payment is not made as described, [ParticipatingProvider] shall be entitled to receive its full billed charges."

Sometimes, however, the payer is not actually responsible for payment, but rather acts as a middleman between the provider and the payer. In those instances, it is essential to create clear lines of accountability. For instance:

"In the event a Payor fails to make payment pursuant to the terms of this Agreement, **[Plan]** shall (a) make such payment on behalf of the Payor, (b) initiate legal action to recover such payment on behalf of **[Participating Provider]**, or (c) assign to the **[Participating Provider]** the right to initiate such action. In the event of (b) or (c), Payor shall provide **[Participating Provider]** a copy of the agreement upon which **[Participating Provider]** may rely in prosecuting such action and shall release **[Participating Provider]** from any further obligation to provide services to **[Members]**."

It is also fairly common for physicians to be denied payment even for patients who were authorized and treated. In addition to requiring the plan to identify members, the following should be helpful in dealing with those instances:

"Verification of coverage at the time of service will be final. Moreover,

notwithstanding any provision of this Agreement to the contrary, any

preauthorized admission or covered service shall be paid, regardless of

any subsequent benefits determination."

Indemnification provisions continue to be troubling in many contracts. First, they tend to be overbroad. Second, they often apply to the doctor and not to the plan. Third, they can jeopardize professional liability insurance coverage. As a general rule, indemnification provisions that apply equally to the parties are considered to be reasonable. For instance, consider:

"To the extent not covered by insurance and subject to the terms and conditions set forth herein, each party (the "Indemnifying Party") agrees to indemnify and hold harmless the other party (the "Indemnified Party") from and against any and all liabilities, damages, claims, deficiencies, assessments, losses, suits, proceedings, actions, investigations, penalties, interest, costs, and expenses, including, without limitation, reasonable fees and expenses of counsel (whether suit is instituted or not and, if instituted, whether at trial or appellate levels) (collectively the "Liabilities"), arising from or in connection with any (i) breach or violation by the Indemnifying Party of any of the obligations, covenants or agreements of the Indemnifying Party contained in this Agreement or (ii) the Indemnifying Party's negligence or willful misconduct."

Fighting the Payer

If, notwithstanding one's best efforts to obtain clarity and fairness, a contract goes bad, there are three provisions in particular that will help or hurt pursuing a claim against a payer: (1) a prevailing party's attorney's fees provision, (2) an arbitration provision and (3) a choice of venue provision.

Prevailing party's fees provisions can be just as harmful as they can be helpful since they help the party that wins a dispute. Nevertheless, in the common situation where the physician has not been paid according to the contract, a prevailing party's fee provision can be invaluable because it gives a lawyer an incentive to take the case, even when there are not a lot of lost fees involved. Here is a fairly simple one:

"Notwithstanding any obligation specified in this Agreement for the participating provider to hold the Payer harmless, in the event of any controversy arising under or relating to the interpretation or implementation of this Agreement or any breach thereof, the prevailing party shall be entitled to payment for all costs and attorneys' fees (both trial and appellate) incurred in connection therewith."

Though arbitration provisions are considered by many to be a "kinder, gentler" alternative to litigation, many detractors think arbitration has become more and more like litigation. On the other hand, depending on the provision, it can unfairly place the dispute within the payer's control and thereby deprive the physician of his or her right to seek redress through litigation. That is, arbitration in the context of payers often turns out to be a fruitless exercise for providers. Moreover, a contract with an arbitration provision cannot generally be the basis of class action litigation, an increasingly popular form of litigation for providers seeking redress from payers.

Nevertheless, if an arbitration provision cannot be negotiated out of the contract, there are some things to watch out for. If, for instance, there is only one arbitrator, it should be one the physician agrees on. Ideally, however, there should be a system for selecting arbitrators that involves each party picking one and the two picking a neutral third. Finally, the arbitrators should apply applicable law and (where possible) the terms of the agreement. One provision that addresses the latter issue is:

"In the event of arbitration pursuant to this Agreement, the arbitrators shall follow controlling law and must (wherever possible) follow the provisions of this Agreement."

Conclusion

Managed care contracts are complex, and the more complicated the situation is (risk contracts, for example), the more that is involved in making the contract precise and fair. Nevertheless, providers will be frustrated to learn that payers are not often responsive to such issues. In this context, size often matters, in the sense that organizations that control the market are far more likely to have meaningful contract negotiations. Still, providers should persist, individually and through their professional societies, in asking for changes that make sense.

In summary, this chapter covered the political nuances of hospital privileges and managed care. Also, we discussed the pitfalls associated with signing the wrong managed care contract. Lastly, we provided some warning signs within a contract that should be removed before signing. In the next chapter, we will discuss employees and their job descriptions. We will also cover contracts and payroll.

EMPLOYEES, CONTRACTS, AND PAYROLL

The first few employees you hire should be for these key positions: front office receptionists, back office clinical assistant (nurse or medical assistant), and a bookkeeper/ billing person/accounts payable/accounts receivable position. One person may be able to serve all these roles at first.

You may not need or be able to afford an office manager from day one. The better office managers are more expensive. Also, if you are not seeing many patients in the beginning, then you might choose to serve in this role. One advantage to this approach is the experience you will gain while serving in that role.

As soon as you start seeing more than five to ten patients a day, your time is more productive seeing patients. Your value is not in micromanagement. It is in seeing patients and doing procedures. Designate an office manager or staff member to help you with all administrative and personnel issues. The experience you gained initially as office manager will prove invaluable when managing this employee's performance.

Job descriptions are an important part of every medical practice. Job descriptions protect you. They help you in the event that an employee is not performing according to his or her job description. There is less confusion upon termination.

Job descriptions also help employees understand their role, to whom they report, and what is expected of them. There should be no ambiguity regarding your employees' roles and responsibilities. Their job descriptions, along with other responsibilities, should be part of their employee handbook. You should have every employee sign an employee handbook and receipt of their job description.

Your front office receptionist is the "face" of the practice. He or she greets your patients, answers the phone, and schedules appointments. He or she is the public's first interaction with your practice. He or she must represent you well. He or she should smile and always be pleasant. He or she should also have the ability to be firm with difficult patients. He or she should be an expert in customer service.

Table 4. The job description for front office receptionist should include these roles and responsibilities:

1. Answering the phone

2. Greeting patients

3. Discharging patients

4. Entering patient information into the computer or chart

5. Cleaning and organizing waiting room in the morning, at lunch, and at close of day

6. Receiving payments from patients and entering into bookkeeping system

7. Managing uniform issues, if you want staff to wear uniforms

8. Keeping track of days and hours worked

9. Pulling patient charts for the day

10. Replacing patient charts at the end of day

11. Cleaning and organizing front office at end of day

12. Preparing day sheet (patients seen with charges and collections) at close of day

13. Reports to: office manager

The back office clinical assistant may be a nurse or a "medical assistant." A medical assistant is less expensive than a nurse. You can train the medical assistant to help you in the manner that you specifically need. If your specialty requires a nurse or your practice is busy enough to support a nurse's salary, then this becomes a viable option.

Table 5. The job description for a back office clinical person should include these roles and responsibilities:

1. Answering the phone when front office receptionist cannot

2. Greeting patients and escorting patients back to the exam rooms

3. Escorting patients from exam room to discharge

4. Taking patient history and assisting with record keeping and medical record charting (either paper or electronic)

5. Performing lab functions, including phlebotomy on patients when indicated

6. Keeping QA (Quality Assurance) and QC (Quality Control) logs and following up all lab and study results

7. Calling patients with study results and physician's plan of action

8. Entering patient information into the computer or chart

9. Cleaning, organizing, and preparing exam room in the morning and before and after patient visits

10. Sterilizing all instruments

11. Managing all medical waste for the office according to office protocols

12. Managing uniform issues if you want staff to wear uniforms

13. Keeping track of days and hours worked

14. Pulling patient charts for the day

15. Replacing patient charts at the end of day

16. Assisting physician or physician extender with all exam room visits and procedures

17. Reports to office manager.

Another position you will need to hire must fill the role of bookkeeper, billing person, and office manager. In the early days of your practice, one person may serve all of these roles. These position types may be dependent upon your own personal preferences. For instance, in the beginning, when I first started my practice, I served as the bookkeeper, payroll administrator, and office manager. I remember every two weeks calculating payroll and paying all the bills myself. Those days are long gone now, but they taught me how to do all those jobs. This knowledge is invaluable. The best use of your time is seeing patients and generating revenue. The savvy medical entrepreneur recognizes this early in the practice development.

Table 6. The job descriptions for bookkeeper and billing personnel/office manager should include these roles and responsibilities (initially this job may be one person):

1. Managing account payables

2. Managing account receivables

3. Using bookkeeping software

4. Reconciling day sheet

5. Ensuring all collections and accounts receivable are reviewed weekly or daily

6. Managing staff and payroll responsibilities

7. Ensuring staff are meeting their roles and responsibilities

8. Having quarterly reviews with staff and reviewing and documenting their performance

9. Setting work schedules and holiday schedules for all staff

10. Ensuring back office personnel are maintaining all logs and manuals

11. Ensuring all billing is being done promptly and accurately

12. Ensuring practice is keeping all compliance manuals and certifications up to date

13. Managing HIPAA, Red Flags Rule, CLIA (Clinical Laboratory Improvement Amendments), and OSHA (Occupational Safety and Health Administration) compliance

14. Recording and maintaining all doctors' CME (Continuing Medical Education) credits

15. Payroll responsibilities (optional)

16. Interfacing with insurance companies to ensure payment for services is as contracted

17. Reports to physician

THE EMPLOYMENT AGREEMENT

Create an employment agreement before you hire your first employee. An attorney should draft or review the agreement. Ask the attorney if you can use the agreement as a template for repeat hiring of nonphysician positions in your practice. You should not have to go back to the attorney every time you have a rehire. A less expensive option is to find prewritten templates. You can find template employment agreements for lower-level positions online or at office supply stores for a few dollars.

In some states you may use an "at-will employment letter" to hire most of your nonprofessional staff. This letter should not be used when you hire a physician. At-will employment letters reflect the following general terms:

1. Compensation
2. Holidays, vacation, sick time, and retirement
3. Termination at will without cause

Before terminating any employee, you should make certain that you have well-documented reasons. Be sure you have had meetings with the employee and have cited him or her for problems with his or her work. Give the employee notice to correct the problems and warn him or her that you may terminate him or her if the problems are not corrected. There are some clear-cut scenarios where an employee breaches his or her employment responsibilities.

In this scenario you can terminate immediately. Those situations are less common.

Make sure every employee signs an employee handbook. The handbook should contain practice policies, procedures, and job descriptions. If you use a payroll company such as ADP or Paychex, the company will help you write your employee handbook, practice policies, and procedures. You can customize this book to your preferences.

There are a few items that may be unique to your practice that you want to include in your practice handbook. Be certain your employees agree not to disparage your name and your practice after termination. This is particularly important with the potential damage a disgruntled employee could cause your reputation. The Internet makes this very easy for disgruntled employees. Be sure your employees agree to protect confidentialities of your patients. All employees must sign all HIPAA policies and Red Flags Rules where indicated.

THE PAYROLL

At the beginning of my practice, I performed the payroll duty myself. I remember calculating each employee's wages every two weeks. This took effort. I would often stress about it. I remember doing payroll at night at home. It's a lot to worry about after taking care of patient care responsibilities. It was an obligation, yet it taught me to understand the costs of payroll and the accompanying taxes. Nonetheless, the time I spent doing this could have been better spent generating revenue for the practice. The cost of a payroll service is nominal and worth the expense. If you really want to hold costs down and there are fewer than five employees, you may do your own payroll. I don't recommend it, though.

You will eventually be delegating the role of performing payroll to someone else. However, as the owner you must pay the payroll taxes. You should understand what this means. Payroll tax is the tax that the corporation must pay whenever it pays wages to employees. FICA is the Federal Income Contribution Act tax and represents the employer's and employee's share of the Social Security tax and the Medicare tax. In the last few years, for example, the employee's share of Social Security is 6.2 percent up to a salary of $106,800, and for the Medicare tax, the employee's share is 1.45 percent of wages with no limit. The employer is responsible for an additional and separate 6.2 percent Social Security tax and 1.45 percent Medicare tax on wages. In some states, employers may be required to withhold state, county, or city income tax. Employers are required to pay state and federal unemployment tax. This means that any salary paid to the shareholder subjects the corporation to payroll taxes such as Social Security and Medicare tax on that salary.

Payroll taxes are avoided for the corporation when shareholders receive distributions. You should not pay a wage earner or employee who is also a shareholder with distributions to avoid salary taxes. Their salary must be reasonable and comparable with other salaries for wage earners in similar positions. Distributions are typically reserved for profits after the salary has been paid.

As your practice grows, you should consider a payroll service or a PEO (Professional Employer Organization). In a PEO, the practice enters into an agreement with the PEO to establish a relationship between you, your employees, and the PEO. You and the PEO become co-employers, instead of the traditional employer and employee relationship. This relationship allows the PEO to help you with employment administration assistance. The PEO shares in many of the employer liabilities. The PEO takes responsibility for Human Resources (HR) administration and compliance. Your employees continue to work at the practice location. You continue to maintain control over your business, but you are relieved of many of the administrative tasks that accompany having employees.

The PEO assumes your employees as theirs for payroll, liability, and benefits purposes. PEOs provide many additional cost benefits, such as better rates on insurance and retirement benefits. A PEO is not totally liability free, and I would recommend considering only the largest PEOs in the country. However, they can be extremely beneficial as you add more and more employees. PEOs are a cost-effective move that will help you to grow your practice.

THE PHYSICIAN CONTRACT

Contracts for physicians should be prepared and reviewed by a board-certified health care attorney. There are many complex health care statutes that must be understood. Issues include noncompete clauses, nonsolicitation clauses, and various regulatory issues that require attention, such as anti-kickback statutes, Stark laws, False Claims Act, Fraud Enforcement Recovery Act, and Health Insurance Portability and Accountability Act (HIPAA).

Noncompete clauses restrict a terminated physician employee from practicing within a certain geographic distance of your practice. This will protect you from the physician soliciting your patients. The noncompete clause must be reasonable; otherwise, it will not be enforceable. You cannot restrict a physician from practicing in an entire state. That restriction is too broad and would not be enforceable. Discuss with your attorney what distance would be reasonable given your situation. Additionally, you can add a liquidated damages clause for noncompetes. This gives you the option of setting a price to forego enforcing the noncompete clause.

Nonsolicitation clauses refer to restricting the act of soliciting patients or employees from a practice at which a physician or other staff member was employed. This is important, as you do not want an employee or physician to be able to solicit your employees away from your practice in the event of termination.

The anti-kickback statute (AKS) results from amendments to the Medicare and Medicaid Anti-Fraud and Abuse Act and makes it illegal to knowing and willfully solicit, receive, offer, or receive payment of any remuneration for referring patients or arranging for acquisition of goods or services reimbursable by Medicare or Medicaid. Violations are punishable by a fine of up to $25,000 and up to five years imprisonment. Additionally, exclusion from federally funded health care programs such as Medicare and Medicaid may result.

Regulatory issues include the Stark laws. These laws protect against physicians referring to a lab or facility that they may have a financial interest in. The law was written to prohibit physicians from making a referral to an entity for the furnishing of designated health services paid by Medicare or Medicaid when the physician or his or her family has a direct or indirect financial relationship with the entity. There are a number of safe harbors within this complex law. Your attorney should help draft your contract to ensure you are not violating any Stark Laws.

The false statements relating to health care matters portion of HIPAA prohibits the making of false statement in any matter involving a health care benefit program.

The contract will need to detail financial responsibility for purchasing a malpractice policy. It will detail limits for malpractice. There are two types of malpractice policies: Claims Made and Occurrence. The Claims Made policy will only respond if the claim is made while the policy is in effect, while with an Occurrence policy, the carrier is responsible for the claim if the incident occurred anytime during the active policy period. If a Claims Made policy is terminated, then continued coverage ("tail") should be purchased until such time that all possible claims that can be brought has expired. The employment contract should define who is responsible for purchasing "tail" coverage.

Additionally, there will be conditions for full-time employment that must be specified in any contract. These conditions include obligations such as obtaining the appropriate licensure to practice medicine and prescribe medications. Physicians must affirm that no medical board has disciplined them and that their license has not been revoked or suspended. They should affirm that they have not been treated or sanctioned for alcohol or substance abuse.

General contract matters that must be considered include the term of the contract. This is often two to three years. Renewal should occur automatically at the end of the term. Termination clauses with and without cause should be defined.

Incentive bonuses in the form of compensation or stock may be considered. Commonly, the physician may receive a bonus based upon revenue generated above a certain amount. This number may tie to the office overhead formula. For instance, assume a 50 percent office overhead and a physician's annual salary of $150,000. The physician may receive an additional 25 percent to 50 percent of revenue generated after he or she has generated $400,000 in revenue. In this scenario, the practice theoretically makes approximately $100,000 on the first $400,000 generated (revenue – overhead – physician salary/package = practice net). Any additional amounts over that $400,000 generated, the physician and the practice share in an agreed-upon percentage.

Table 7. Important points that need to be covered in the contract with a physician:

1. Realistic and reasonable noncompete clauses.

2. Liquidation clauses for noncompete.

3. Malpractice issues regarding their responsibility for tail coverage.

4. Obligations, duties, and responsibilities for your practice.

5. Definition of the on-call schedule.

6. Definition of the necessity for maintaining hospital privileges.

7. Definition of bonuses, salary, and productivity requirements.

8. If you are going to offer a partnership track, define the terms.

9. Be certain nothing in the contract violates the Stark laws, anti-kickback statutes, and HIPAA.

10. Clarify that you own the patients' records in the event of termination.

11. Include a termination without cause with thirty-day notice.

12. Define who will pay for CME (Continuing Medical education) credits.

13. Define how many days will be paid for attending a professional meeting per year.

14. Define how much you will pay for licensure for boards, tests, exams, DEA license, medical society memberships, dues, accreditation for hospitals, and hospital staff fees.

15. Include a clause for nonsolicitation of employees.

STAT CONSULT FROM JEFF COHEN, BOARD-CERTIFIED HEALTH CARE ATTORNEY

No one speaks directly to physicians who are new in practice, and there are basic things you must know before you step into the world as a practicing physician.

First, not to be cynical, but many people in business see physicians as income opportunities. When you go into practice, you will be inundated with offers and opportunities, all of which need to be carefully scrutinized. The key, for purposes of this book, is for you to be armed with knowledge.

The three primary areas of knowledge you must have are (1) liability for fraud and abuse (including self referral prohibitions), (2) what to look out for in an employment opportunity, and (3) where to seek legal advice.

Fraud and Abuse

Fraud and abuse laws encompass several key state and federal laws, such as the Anti-kickback Statute, the Stark laws, and (in Florida) the Florida Patient Self-referral Law of 1992. Additionally, many states have their own versions of the federal kickback and referral prohibitions. The core concept to keep in mind is that it is illegal for you to pay or be paid anything (not just money—even gifts) in exchange for referring patients. For instance, a home health company or medical device supplier may approach you and say, "Hey, if you send patients to us or use our products, we'll make you a medical director or consultant and pay you money each month." Get advice right away! Such arrangements can be entered into if there is a legitimate purpose and the arrangement is documented to comply with key laws. Generally speaking, if compensation and referrals are spoken about in the same sentence, you are on shaky ground and need to get advice immediately!

Being paid for patient referrals is illegal and will subject you to both criminal and civil monetary penalties. Moreover, there is settled case law that, even if one purpose of your business arrangement is to compensate you for patient referrals and the rest of the business arrangement is permissible, you are in deep water and subject to fines and imprisonment. That said, there are ways to be appropriately paid for necessary and appropriate medical services, including for providing medical director services. Some of the regulatory requirements include, for instance:

1. the agreement has to be for necessary services;

2. it has to be written and specifically describe what you are to do;

3. it must be for a period of at least twelve months;

4. compensation has to be set in advance and not vary based on the value or volume of business generated between the parties;

5. compensation must be consistent with fair market value, as defined in the relevant laws.

Self-referral restrictions are pretty clear at the federal level, but vary greatly from state to state. When people refer to "Stark," they are generally referring to the self-referral aspect, though there is a separate section of that law that pertains to financial relationships between health care providers. Generally speaking, the self-referral restrictions pertain to (1) you or your immediate family having any ownership interest or financial relationship with certain health care services providers, and (2) you or your immediate family members referring to that provider. The sorts of services that are caught by the prohibition are generally defined as "designated health services" (DHS) and include such things as PT, rehab, clinical lab, home health, and diagnostic imaging services. Since those definitions change from time to time, you will need help to determine which services fall within the definition. If the person or entity you are going to refer to provides DHS services, check with counsel to see if you have a prohibited relationship with the provider of such services. The laws have many exceptions (e.g., the "in-office ancillary services exception" for "group practices"), and care is needed to ensure compliance.

One of the other key aspects of the fraud and abuse laws that should be easy to keep in mind is that nearly every business arrangement you may enter into (e.g., leases, employment, etc.) must be encompassed in a written agreement, and the contents of the agreement are governed by federal and sometimes state law! You can lease a car on any term imaginable, but if you enter into a lease on a percentage basis, you may be breaking the fraud and abuse laws. Health care business transactions *are strictly regulated by state and federal law. Even how much you are paid and how you are paid for the services you provide is regulated. Though the nuances and legal issues are too numerous to treat in a comprehensive way, suffice it to say that you will need expert advice navigating those waters.*

Employment Agreements

As a new physician, you very likely will be offered employment. First rule: if it isn't in writing, it isn't binding on the parties. Everything that is important to you must be contained in a written agreement. And what sorts of things should you look for?

Details about your work. Where will you be working? Can the employer move you around too much? What about call? How much call are you required to cover? What are your office hours? Do you require any special personnel or equipment to do your job? The contract must be as specific as possible about what your duties and responsibilities are.

The length of the contract. Most contracts are for an initial period of twelve months. That said, they can often be terminated by either party with thirty to ninety days' written notice.

Noncompetes. In some states, like Florida, noncompetition provisions are common. And you should assume they are enforceable! The key things to look for are how long they last (usually up to two years following termination), how big the geographic radius is, and what services you are prohibited from performing. Some negotiating points include:

- *Seeing if they will agree to a short "honeymoon" period, where the noncompete does not apply;*

- *Seeing if they will reduce the durational or geographic scope;*

- *Ensuring it only applies to what you do and to competitors like your employer, not a broad prohibition of practicing medicine in any way for anyone;*

- *Seeing if the employer will create exceptions (1) if you are terminated without cause, (2) if you terminate for cause, and (3) if they do not renew the contract;*

- *Finally, remember that if you are joining a practice via a hospital-assisted recruitment agreement, the contract may not contain a noncompete. The thing to keep in mind about noncompetes is that, even if you think you ought to be entitled to break one, and you win, it will cost you lots of money and take a lot longer to resolve than you may think. Take them seriously!*

Malpractice insurance. The sorts of malpractice insurance policies and costs vary greatly from state to state. Basically there are two types: (1) Claims Made, and (2) Occurrence. Claims Made policies will only cover you if the claim is made at the time the insurance is in effect (and the claim pertains to the period when you were insured by the specific insurer). Occurrence coverage applies even if the claim is made after the policy is cancelled before the claim is made. In Florida, for instance, nearly all policies are written in a Claims Made form. First, make sure the contract covers you for malpractice claims. Second, if you are insured under a Claims Made policy, then you may want "tail" coverage when the contract expires or is terminated. Tail coverage is an extra policy that can be bought which extends the period of time the policy is in effect beyond the time the contract expires or is terminated. For instance, if the Claims Made policy is in effect for all of 2010, but then you go to work for a new employer, effective January 1, 2011, the insurer of the new employer will not cover you for the claims arising in connection with your prior employer, and the insurer of your prior employer will not cover you either unless "tail" insurance is purchased within a short time after you leave your prior employer. And it's expensive, so you will want to negotiate (1) it being provided for you, and (2) who pays for it at the time you negotiate your employment contract.

Compensation. The contract needs to be clear about what you are paid. Normally you will receive a flat annual salary and productivity compensation. Rather than being generally referred to in the contract, the productivity compensation ought to be specifically described. As far as bonuses go, there are hundreds of formulas, but generally, you can expect to receive something once the practice has received about twice as much as your base compensation.

Partnership. Ideally, the contract should say when you get to be a partner and how much you have to pay to be one (or what the formula is). It is common, however, for new employees not to be provided much in the way of details.

Here are some secrets you need to know about contracting:

1. Don't be afraid to ask for what you want. The employer is a businessperson. New doctors are sometimes afraid to ask for what they want because they are afraid the

> *employer will back out. Don't be afraid to ask. Just ask respectfully.*
>
> 2. *It takes a while to generate revenue. It can take months to get on managed care panels and care for those patients. It can take a while to get added to the group's Medicare group provider number. Get these things started early on. And remember that if you are counting on income for bonus purposes, etc., the first three months show generally very low income.*

In summary, this chapter covered hiring employees and physician employees. We covered the contract issues for both types of employees. We touched upon some of the regulations that impact hiring physicians such as Stark laws, malpractice issues, and noncompete issues. We also discussed payroll, payroll taxes, and payroll service companies. In the next chapter, we discuss billing options. We cover the pros and cons of hiring an outside billing company versus billing internally. We also explain the basics of billing.

BILLING AND GETTING PAID

Billing is the process of submitting a claim for a patient encounter. It requires entering a code for the procedure performed by a provider (CPT or Current Procedural Terminology code) during a patient encounter and matching that code to a diagnosis code (ICD or International Classification of Diseases code). These codes are then grouped together along with a fee, and a claim is generated.

Computer software does most, if not all, of this for you. There are several good programs. These are called practice management software. They are frequently bundled into or alongside electronic health record (EHR) software.

After you generate a bill for a patient encounter, the bill is submitted electronically via an electronic CMS (Centers for Medicare and Medicaid services) 1500 form (formerly HCFA or Health Care Financing and Administration form). That bill is sent directly to the patient's insurance company. This is the first part of the billing process.

The second part of the billing process is referred to as posting payment. Most insurers will post automatically and electronically to the patient's financial record. Posting is performed within the practice management software program. This is a huge savings for your practice. However, posting manually is required for noninsurance payments and for some secondary insurers. Secondary insurance is insurance that covers the remainder of a patient's bill after the primary insurer has met its financial obligations.

The last part of the billing process is the collection of fees and managing accounts receivable. This is the most time-consuming part of billing. It requires diligence to make sure your receivables don't get out of control. You will need to regularly monitor your 30/60/90/120 day receivables. You will need to have a staff person responsible for billing patients for the balances due after their insurance payments (called "balance billing"). Additionally, you will need to send bills, collect payments, and post these payments manually. It is important to understand that most insurance companies' payments will post automatically to your billing software. Balance billing to secondary insurances and patients will likely require personnel and time.

There are pros and cons to billing internally versus outsourcing your billing to a billing company. I have done it both ways and was most happy when billed internally. I found that the billing company required much of my staff's time just to check and make sure they didn't make mistakes. It made many mistakes that would not have been detected had we not checked on them. I prefer to do my own billing rather than outsource it.

Table 8. Pros and Cons of billing internally (without billing service).

Pros:

1. In the beginning you will be slow enough to watch the billing and to hire the one staff member that can bill.

2. If you do it yourself initially, you will learn all about billing issues. If you ever switch to a billing company, you will be able to monitor its production.

3. Self-billing is simpler these days. Almost everything is computerized. Most of the posting of insurance payments is done automatically.

4. There are excellent billing software programs that are inexpensive. I prefer a hosted ASP (Application Service Provider) solution. You don't have to load or maintain software locally on your own computers (servers). ASP systems are Web based and very secure. I highly recommend ASP models.

5. You have complete control over your billing and your accounts receivable (AR), and your staff talks directly to your patients about their balances due. Billing companies may be rude to your patients, hassle patients, or not answer customer service questions promptly. Hence, your staff dealing with your patients is a good choice.

Cons:

1. You have to hire trained personnel to perform this function.

2. The AR and collection portion can be overwhelming and may require hiring additional personnel to support the growth of your practice.

3. May limit your ability to grow and add more doctors since you will need to add more employees.

4. You have to purchase a practice management billing software program and maintain and support it.

Table 9. Pros and Cons of outsourcing to a billing company:
Pros

1. The work is outsourced, so you can focus on your patients and grow your core business.

2. You do not have to hire personnel to perform this function.

3. You do not have to buy or maintain billing software.

4. In the beginning of your practice, you may not have the expertise or resources to do billing internally.

Cons:

1. Billing companies may provide bad customer service and thus reflect poorly on you and your practice.

2. Billing companies may make many mistakes, so you have to be prepared for this by hiring someone to check on them.

3. Billing companies may be difficult to deal with because they are offsite.

4. If the billing company does something wrong, such as overbill a patient, you are still liable.

5. Billing companies are only as good as the lower-level employees they hire. They probably pay those people less than someone you would find.

6. Billing companies are difficult to break away from once you have started with them.

7. They are often very expensive, despite what they show and tell you.

PITFALLS TO AVOID

Before you contract with a billing company, review its termination policy carefully. Make sure you can terminate without cause and without any penalty at any time. Make sure all the records and billing records are yours and will be returned to you.

PEARL

You should negotiate with billing companies. They will quote that the average fee is 6 percent on collections. I have found that most billing companies will negotiate and will accept 4 percent.

After I discovered that our billing company was making many billing mistakes, I decided to terminate the contract. This is not easy. Make sure you read the termination provisions in your contract carefully. I realized that I had to play hardball with our billing company. It had made many costly mistakes. These were financial errors that cost us thousands of dollars. The company provided poor customer service. It created unnecessary liability by making billing errors that were not caused by us. I knew I had to change. I decided to do the billing internally and use hosted ASP solution for billing. My costs would drop significantly.

The problem was how I could terminate the contract. The company required a minimum sixty-day notice. This meant that I would have to pay it for at least sixty more days. I could not stomach paying it another penny since it had cost me so much in billing mistakes. My other concern was how I would get all my patient records, data, and balances transferred over and back to us. The accounts receivable would be a nightmare to transfer over. I did not want the company to know I was terminating it. I needed it to continue to bill for us until I was ready to take it over. There were hundreds of thousands of dollars in billings per month and accounts receivables.

I decided I would not send it any new patient bills. I hoped that it would not notice. If it asked, I would say that we were on vacation or that our staff was behind. I would not pay any bill that I owed it. That was the only leverage I had. Two months elapsed before the company noticed that I had not paid it. I owed a significant amount. I gave it immediate notice for termination and that it had breached its obligations. Of course, it did not accept this. The company informed me that since I terminated its services, I had to pay it a termination fee equal to sixty days of billing. This was over $20,000. I was prepared for this. I disagreed, politely, and reminded the company that I had scratched this clause out of the contract before I signed it. And, furthermore, it breached its obligations, so I was terminating it for cause. It was not due any termination fee. The lesson here is to hold firm. It is sometimes easy for a doctor to "roll over." We are so busy with patients that we are not prepared for fights. I was. You will be, too, after reading this. I informed the company that it could sue me for what it perceived I owed. I told it that I would make every doctor in our county aware of how bad its service was. I explained that I would settle with the company for an amount less than what we owed it excluding any termination fee. I explained that if we settled upon a fair amount, then I would release funds only upon receiving full backups of all our data.

The company had a choice: sue me for a termination fee and risk other doctors learning about our problems, or accept a settlement fee. It called me back asking for a settlement. It would waive its claim for any termination or penalties. We received everything we needed, and I paid the company a fair amount. You can see that this process is not easy. It is stressful. You must understand what you are getting into when you sign up with a billing service.

In summary, this chapter covered the three critical components of getting paid in your practice: billing, posting, and collecting. We analyzed the pros and cons of billing internally or outsourcing to a billing company. Lastly, we discussed what to watch out for when contracting with or terminating a third=party billing company. In the next chapter, we will uncover the truths about office software, electronic health records, and technology for the practice.

TECHNOLOGY AND THE ELECTRONIC HEALTH RECORDS FOR THE OFFICE

I have worked with EHR (electronic health records) companies for the last ten years. I helped a small company called Medinotes with its clinical templates. Medinotes was recently acquired by a public EHR company called Eclypsis. I created and founded one of the first personal health record (PHR) companies, PassportMD. This was five years before President Obama began talking about it. It was years before Microsoft and Google released their versions. PassportMD was acquired in 2009. Lastly and most importantly I purchased an EHR for my practice many years ago. I understand the headaches of owning, setting up, installing, and maintaining an EHR for a medical practice.

If I were writing this book three years ago, I would have said wait five more years before you purchase an EHR. However, in the last two years, President Obama has put the electronic health records industry front and center for doctors. If you are in any sort of practice today, this must now be a consideration. Although there are still no mandates to adopt EHRs, there are stimulus funds available for doctors. The stimulus funds are available through the American Recovery and Reinvestment Act (ARRA) of 2009. Eligible practices must participate in Medicare and Medicaid.

The practice's EHR must be used in a "meaningful" way (we will discuss this definition later).

I started shopping for EHR programs ten years ago. It was very different then. There were many more small companies and more choices. The larger companies today acquired many of the smaller companies. I was an early adopter of technology and wanted an EHR for my practice. I compared prices and features. I found the most user-friendly and least expensive system. After purchasing, installing, and using the software, I quickly learned that the least expensive component of owning an EHR is the initial software purchase. These additional costs include the cost of additional hardware, networking equipment, third-party software, and recurrent software licensing fees.

The most significant cost that physicians overlook is the cost of an IT (information technology) consultant to support the systems in the office. Most physicians, including me, are not very knowledgeable about networking. I had to hire a computer consultant to manage my networks, maintain my hardware, install software updates, and schedule all backups. The computer consultant or IT (information technology) consultant is affectionately referred to as our "IT guy." IT consultants are readily available. Good ones can be difficult to find. You need to ask around. Ask other doctors that have computerized practices for referrals. Hiring the wrong IT consultant can be disastrous.

My first IT consultant was great for the first few years he worked for us. He was smart, hardworking, and trustworthy. He worked for several other physician colleagues. However, after a few years of service, I noticed that his monthly bills were becoming disproportionately higher than prior months. His bills no longer accurately reflected the amount of time that he spent working on our practice. He started to bill us to fix things that he did wrong or that he "broke." I started noticing a different level of attention. Coincidentally, one of my physician colleagues that also contracted with him called me to see if I had noticed a change in his performance. She was having problems, too. I realized that I had to make a change. This was not easy. It was further complicated because we had a dispute over balances due. I was scared to argue with him because he had access to all of our computers and our operations. I was nervous that he would do something malicious to our systems. He had access and the passwords. He could easily corrupt files, crash our systems, or change our passwords. You have to be very careful to select an IT person that you can trust and that won't be malicious when you part. You can never be too certain, but try to protect against this scenario. The best way to minimize your vulnerability is to control all master passwords. Be certain you are the administrator for all the passwords and have master privileges. Privileges are assigned along with passwords. They define who can see certain applications or who can change certain system settings. Regardless, whatever precautions you take, you are still vulnerable. I was lucky. I was able to terminate our relationship and reach a settlement on the outstanding balance. He did not act maliciously. Some months later, I ran into one of his former employees. He told me the consulting business had closed shortly after we terminated. He was suing his former boss, our IT consultant, for back pay.

The key characteristics of a good IT consultant are reliability, integrity, and experience. Networks and computer systems crash all the time. It is unpredictable, but inevitably networks crash in the middle of the busiest patient day. You need someone who is always willing and able to tend to your practice in an emergency. Spell this out in any arrangement. I pay my current IT consultant a flat monthly retainer for support of my computers and networks. Most consultants charge based upon the number of hardware systems and networks they are responsible for. Get a quote from a few different providers and compare this number with references. Remember, do not sign any support contract unless you are able to terminate at any time without penalty and without cause.

My initial fears with incorporating electronic health records into my practice was losing saved patient data. I think many doctors share this concern. My fear was validated one morning when I arrived at the office to find that no one could access any patient data. We could not see our patients' schedules, billing, or patient charts. I had spent a lot of money creating a system of redundancy.

Redundancy means that the system backs up a mirror image of one hard drive to another server. We had two additional servers that served this purpose. So, redundancy was in triplicate. If one server failed, we could retrieve information from the second redundant server. If the second server crashed simultaneously, which seemed highly unlikely, we had a third server to retrieve the information from.

As luck would have it, two of my servers crashed simultaneously. I thought, no problem, we would get the information we needed from our third server. However, when we went to retrieve the data off the third server, it appeared that our regularly scheduled backups were not reaching the third server. Our IT consultant was supposed to be monitoring this. It had been months since our third server had current data. At this point, I was livid.

My IT consultant told me we would have one chance to retrieve the data. We could send the first server to a catastrophic recovery service. These are the same companies that work for the government retrieving highly confidential data off corrupted computer systems. They charge $20,000 whether or not they get the data back. We had no choice. I sent the server to the company overnight and within a day had all my data back. I found out that I had insurance for this type of event. In the end everything worked out.

The lesson I learned from this experience was to make sure that I always monitor my backups. I added an additional remote offsite server to back up data. Make sure you have insurance to cover you for catastrophic data loss. The best way to minimize this risk is to use an ASP system and back up your data locally in the event you have a catastrophic loss.

I spend a minimum of $50,000 annually supporting my software programs, updating software, licensing software and paying an IT consultant to manage and handle these functions for my practice.

An electronic health record is commonly referred to as an EHR. It is the software that is responsible for tracking, monitoring, and charting your patient's health. An EHR, by definition, enables you to input data as well as search for data. A document management system is basically a filing cabinet that allows you to view images of the patient's record. Document management systems do not allow databasing, data searching, or data manipulation. A hybrid EHR combines attributes of both systems. You can input and track data but also manage images. A personal health record or PHR is a patient's record of his or her electronic health information. The PHR is, by definition, carried by the patient. Some EHR programs have PHR attributes so that physicians can create a PHR on behalf of their patient.

There are three main types of software that every practice needs to consider purchasing: practice management software, electronic health records (EHR), and bookkeeping software.

Practice management software does just that: it helps you "manage" your practice. It includes patient check-in and billing software. A few years ago, most practice management systems were stand-alone. They were separate from electronic health record vendors. Practice management software was critical for a practice to function, bill, and collect payments. Electronic health record systems were not critical to the business of the practice. As a result, adoption for practice management software was early. Most insurance providers no longer accept paper claims.

In contrast, even with government incentives, adoption for electronic health records is slow. I believe the incentives for electronic health record adoption are not high enough. The incentives are an important part of accelerating physician adoption. Adoption by a critical mass of physicians is still a function of the strength of the incentives offered. Most electronic health record systems remain difficult to implement. Many doctors are too comfortable with their paper charts. I believe this will change, but incentives must be greater for physicians.

Many EHR vendors now bundle software together so that it contains EHR and practice management applications. The advantage of getting both applications from one vendor is interoperability. Interoperability means that your practice management system will interface seamlessly with your EHR.

I prefer hosted ASP (application service providers) or Web-based systems. It is more costly and difficult to keep the software updated and maintained when it resides on a local server in the office. This is called a server-based EHR system. A Web-based or hosted ASP system is more analogous to a tenant-and-landlord relationship. There are fewer upfront costs, but these may include monthly fees. I have done it both ways and found that the hosted ASP system works better. When I had a server-based EHR system, I had many maintenance headaches. The costs to maintain my servers increased year after year.

I suggest you narrow down your selections to only those vendors that sell hosted ASP systems. These vendors are required by federal law to follow HIPAA (Health Insurance Portability and Accountability Act) and to keep all data confidential and secure. Most vendors will permit you to download patient data at any time. This will help prevent data loss. It will also make sure that you have a second copy of data in the event you terminate with your ASP provider. It is a good idea to have your IT (Information Technology) consultant help you set up a schedule of periodic downloads of your patient data, including demographics, and billing information. This information should be backed up to locally hosted servers or to a remote storage facility.

After you select a vendor, but before you sign any contract, make certain you have the right to terminate "at any time for any reason without any penalty." And make certain that upon termination you are granted full rights and access to download all data related to your practice.

It is much easier to start your practice with an EHR than to go back and do it later. However, if you do choose to do it later, it is not complicated. Most EHR vendors understand the process of converting your paper charts to an EHR. They will help you with conversion.

There are some EHR vendors that are pure "document management" systems. This means that they help you store images of paper, notes, and x-rays. This is similar to the way you may store photos or documents at home on your personal computer. Document management systems may be more practical depending on the workflow and type of practice you will have.

The drawback to a "document management" system is that it is not a "true" EHR. A true EHR enables "databasing" of elements of the patient record. Data is retrievable. This is a critical component of the "meaningful use" definitions.

"Meaningful use," as discussed later in this chapter, is a requirement that must be met by physicians through the use of their EHR to be eligible to receive incentives through the American Recovery and Reinvestment Act (ARRA) of 2009. The government believes that the ability to database elements of the medical record is critical. Elements that would be databased include providers, patient demographics, medications, illnesses, social history, and allergies.

It is generally assumed that databasing will enable greater efficiencies and fewer medical mistakes. This theoretically results in reduced costs. This is the contention by the EHR vendors and by the government. It should be noted that some skeptics and many doctors do not subscribe to this belief. It is interesting to note that those practices that choose pure document management software systems have calculated the cost and benefits. The practice concludes that the return on investment (ROI) for a document management system in terms of practice efficiency, physician effort, and physician time trumps the value of incorporating a "true" EHR. This is despite receiving federal stimulus money for a "true" EHR.

In addition to practice management software and EHR software, there is a need for bookkeeping software. Bookkeeping software helps manage accounts payable, accounts receivable, cash flow, profit and loss, inventory tracking, supplies, and sales of goods in an office.

A well-known example of this type of software is Quickbooks, but there are many others to choose from. Some practice management software programs incorporate a proprietary form of bookkeeping software.

In addition to software, you will need to purchase hardware. The hardware requirements will depend upon the type of practice management, EHR software, and book-keeping software used. Inexpensive desktops in the front office for clerical work are ideal. Physicians may choose laptops, tablets, or desktops to run the EHR. Even with ASP-hosted solutions, you still need to back up work done daily. Backups of data can be done to servers or to less expensive external storage devices.

You will need an IT consultant to help you set up a secure network that all of your computers reside on. This way all the computers on the network can be scheduled to back up regularly to an external hard drive, server, or remote site. A network ensures that everyone is working in the same environment. It enables input on one computer to show up instantaneously on another. Networked computers may be configured to access the ASP (application service provid-ers) software. You can instantly monitor your practice and patients from wherever you are. Gone are the days, when I first started, of carrying around fifty patient charts from one office to another. I have listed in the table below the questions you should ask an EHR vendor before making a purchase.

Table 10. Attributes I recommend confirming before pur-chasing EHR (Electronic Health Record):

1. EHR system should be a hosted ASP software system.

2. EHR should be a hybrid system permitting both document management features and database management templates.

3. Meets the criteria for "meaningful use" (this is an evolving definition, but current information may be found at www.federalregister.gov/inspection.aspx#special). "Meaningful use" implies that federal stimulus funds will be available to you to help offset the cost of EHR software investment. (See next table for partial definition of "meaningful use.")

4. EHR integrates seamlessly with lab software and systems.

5. EHR enables personal health record building option and patient portal.

6. EHR integrates or includes practice management software.

7. EHR integrates and includes scheduling program.

8. EHR vendor is solid and reputable and been in business for more than five years.

9. EHR must be CCHIT certified. This means that the Certification Commission for Health Information Technology (CCHIT) has certified the vendor and the product according to various standards.

10. EHR vendor must be willing and able to download your data to your own servers locally on a regular basis. You must always have access to the data in the event the vendor goes out of business.

11. EHR support always available.

12. EHR ease of use.

13. EHR integrates or supports dictations.

14. Ease of implementing the system in your practice.

15. Ease of customizing the system for your preferences.

16. Confirm that the system can be accessed from anywhere.

17. Confirm that the EHR has attributes particular to your specialty.

18. Confirm that the company has had over one hundred installs, at a minimum.

19. Confirm that the company has over one hundred physician users, at a minimum.

20. Confirm that the EHR company supports the product.

21. Confirm that the EHR vendor will help facilitate receiving federal stimulus incentives.

22. Confirm the total cost of the software system installed and working.

23. Confirm the monthly maintenance costs.

24. Define additional computer hardware needed to purchase.

25. Define additional local networking software needed to purchase.

26. Define how much local networking and hardware support you will need.

27. Define the additional third-party software the vendor requires you to purchase.

28. Define the annual and monthly costs and licensing fees for the third-party software.

Last year Congress approved the Health Information Technology and Economic and Clinical Health Act (HITECH). The HITECH Act authorizes incentive payments to Medicare and Medicaid physicians. The incentive payments may total as much as $44,000 over a four-year period. The goal of the HITECH Act is not only adoption of technology but "meaningful use" of a certified EHR system. "Meaningful use" is defined by a set of very specific criteria. This act also applies to hospitals, but for this book's purpose we will only deal with physicians in private practice. The "most recent" and "final" version of meaningful use criteria has reduced the obligations of practitioners from meeting the twenty-five measures originally proposed. The Centers for Medicare and Medicaid Services (CMS) have revised the criteria, moving away from an "all or nothing" approach to a more graduated approach. The criteria that must now be met in part or in full can be divided into two groups: a set of fifteen "core" objectives that must all be met, and then a "menu" set of ten tasks. Only five of the tasks must be met. The core objectives comprise basic functions that an electronic health record must perform to improve health care and delivery. They are essential elements of a traditional practice and medical chart. Other core objectives focus on improving safety, quality, and efficiency of care. The menu items include such functions as drug formulary checks, submitting information to immunization registries, incorporating lab results, and patient reminders. Additionally, CMS lowered thresholds that have to be met for some of the respective criteria. For instance, the electronic prescribing threshold was reduced from 75 percent to 40 percent of all prescriptions written. I believe that the criteria are still too onerous for most physicians to meet, and I predict that only 20 percent of private practices will meet the criteria to receive the full incentive payment of $44,000. For instance, consecutive years of participation are mandatory, and if a doctor skips one year of participation or does not qualify one year, then he is removed from receiving any payment for that year. If a physician adopts in 2011, he may receive $18,000, then $12,000 in 2012, $8,000 in 2013, $4,000 in 2014, and finally $2,000 in 2015. Doctors seeking incentive payments will also be required to report on clinical quality measures: three required core measures and three additional quality measures from a menu of thirty-eight measures. Many of these criteria remain unrealistic and probably originate from political rhetoric rather than a true desire to help doctors offset the burdens and costs associated with meeting these criteria.

The table below lists the recently revised fifteen core objectives that must be met to be eligible for incentive payments. The table is meant to provide an abbreviated but concise summary reference of the core objectives defined by HITECH. The full description and requirement should be reviewed at www.cms.gov.

Table 11. Fifteen core, required objectives for meaningful use qualifications and menu set of measures for meaningful use (providers must report on five). (Sources: www.federalregister.gov/inspection.aspx #special and R. Chaudhari, "Will I receive stimulus money for adopting an ," *Dermatology World*, September 2010.)

1. Use of computer physician order entry (*must represent 30 percent of all medication orders).

2. Implement drug-drug, drug-allergy, and drug formulary checks.

3. Maintain up-to-date problem list of current and active diagnoses based on ICD-9 or SnoMed CT (*must represent 80 percent of all unique patients).

4. Generate and transmit prescriptions electronically (*must represent 40 percent of all prescriptions).

5. Maintain active medication list (*must represent 80 percent of all unique prescriptions).

6. Maintain active medication allergy list (*must represent 80 percent of all unique patients).

7. Record demographics (*must represent 50 percent of all unique patients).

8. Record vital signs and body mass index (*must represent 50 percent of all unique patients; this requirement has an exception for providers that do not collect vital signs).

9. Record smoking status for patients thirteen years of age or older (*must represent 50 percent of all unique patients; this requirement has an exception for providers that do not see patients thirteen years of age or older).

10. Provide patients with electronic copy of health information upon request (*must represent 50 percent of all unique patients; exception is for providers that do not receive requests).

11. Report ambulatory clinical quality measures.

12. Implement one clinical decision support rules relevant to specialty priority by reporting relevant quality measures to CMS (*required once per reporting period).

13. Provide clinical summaries for patients for each office visit (*required on 50 percent of all office visits; the exception is for those providers that do not have office visits).

14. Capability to exchange key clinical information (*tequired to perform at least one test).

15. Protect electronic health information (*tequired to perform a security risk analysis with security updates).

Menu set of measures for meaningful use

1. Implement drug formulary checks and have access to at least on drug formulary.

2. Incorporate clinical lab-test results to certified EHR technology as structured data (required to represent 40 percent of all lab orders; the exception is for providers who order no lab tests and don't receive a numeric format during EHR reporting period).

3. Generate at least one report listing the patients of the provider with a specific condition (*required once per reporting period).

4. Send reminders to patients per patient preference for preventive care (*must represent 20 percent of all unique patients over sixty-five or under five years of age; the exception is for providers who don t see patients in this age range).

5. Provide patients with timely electronic access to their health information (required on 10 percent of all unique patients).

6. Use certified EHR to identify patient specific education resources (*required on 10 percent of all unique patients).

7. Perform medication reconciliation for patients (required on 50 percent of all transitions of care; the exception is for those providers that do not receive transitions of care).

8. Provide summary of care record for each transition of care or referral (*required on 50 percent of all transitions; the exception is for those providers that do not receive transitions).

9. Capability to submit electronic data to immunization registries (required to perform one test during reporting period; the exception is for those providers who do not administer immunizations).

10. Capability to submit electronic syndromic surveillance data to public health agencies (*required to be performed at least once; the exception is for providers who don't collect reportable syndromic data).

In summary, this chapter covered the critical elements of technology needed for your practice. This included the three types of software every practice needs to consider purchasing: electronic health record (EHR) software, practice management software, and bookkeeping software. We covered the important criteria that an EHR should meet prior to your purchasing the system. We reviewed the need for redundancy of computer systems to protect data. Also, we reviewed the importance of hiring the right IT consultant to help with all technology aspects of the practice. Lastly, we covered the recently released "meaningful use" requirements that your software must meet for you to receive federal stimulus funds. In the next chapter, we will cover how to plan, design, and locate an office.

PLANNING, DESIGNING, AND LOCATING AN OFFICE

Initially, you should enter into a short-term (one- to two-year) lease of office space. Short-term space will be pre-existing, so you will not have much flexibility on the layout. However, if you do have a "buildout" or the opportunity to design the flow of your office, here are a few suggestions:

Be certain that your waiting room has space for enough chairs. Initially you will be slower and will have fewer patients. When I first started, I projected only two or three patients an hour. I had eight chairs in the waiting room. Within two years I had to move offices because I could not accommodate the patients in my waiting room. My next office had only twelve chairs in the waiting room. I outgrew that space in two years. I always had enough examination rooms. However, my waiting room could not accommodate patients, their family, and friends. I had people standing up in the waiting room. This was not acceptable. Be certain of the volume demands on your waiting room before you sign a long-term lease.

> ## Table 12. Formula for calculating the minimum number of chairs you need in the waiting room
>
> A good rule of thumb is take the number of exam rooms that you will have in your office and add the number of chairs in your waiting room, and the total should be 2.5 times the number of patients you schedule per hour (I call this the "Hacker Rule").

If you expect to have four to six patients scheduled per hour, than you really need at least ten to fifteen chairs in the waiting room. The logic behind the Hacker Rule is if you have four patients scheduled in an hour, then four exam rooms accommodate those appointments. Thirty-three percent of patients show up early for their appointments, 33 percent of patients show up on time, and 33 percent show up late. Your on-time patients will occupy the exam rooms, and others will be sitting in your waiting room. You will have "add-ons" or "walk-ins," too. Emergencies occur and will have to be worked into your schedule. Almost all of the patients show up with at least one additional family member. Your waiting room needs to account for these patients and their additional family members.

The design of the office should account for collection of payments. In my practice, we often encountered patients "bolting" out the door so that they did not have to pay their bill. This was easy to do, because I had one staff member checking in and checking out patients. The staff member would be occupied checking in patients and could not "catch" the patients checking out. Many patients "bolted" for the exit without paying their bills. For the ideal traffic flow, you should have a separate check-in or entrance for patients coming for their appointments. You should have a separate checkout or exit after the appointment is complete. This may be ideal, but often you won't have the space for it. However, if you have the opportunity to build out your office space, I suggest you consider this sort of patient flow design. It will decrease congestion during the check-in and check-out process. It will be less likely for your staff to miss collecting payments from your patients. It is better to have one person register patients as they check into your office. You should have a second person check out patients, make their follow-up appointment, and collect payments and co-pays. In the beginning you may only be able to afford one staff member to fill both of these roles. The practice will become busier, and then a second staff person can be hired to check out patients.

Table 13. Follow these suggestions when planning the design of the office and examination rooms.

1. Exam rooms should have space for one exam table, one to two chairs for additional family members, one stool on rollers for you, one small work station desk, and a computer. Ideally, there should be one sink in each room.

2. Depending upon your specialty, you may need a room for labs and blood draws. You may also need a room for procedures or diagnostic tests.

3. Depending upon your specialty, you may need a room for your nurses and medical assistants to do their charting and work.

4. You should have one bathroom for patients, one bathroom for staff, and ideally one bathroom for physicians. If you can't have this many bathrooms, staff and physicians should share one bathroom.

5. You will need one office for physicians (I would suggest sharing offices among physicians instead of having an executive office for each physician).
6. You will need an additional small space to house your computers, hard drives, and servers.

THE OFFICE SPACE

When I first started practicing, I shared space with another doctor. He was a cardiologist. This was a great short-term approach. It gave me a year to learn what I needed and wanted for office space. I grew out of this situation and bought my own office. I do suggest starting small rather than buying a large office. The temptation is always to buy a larger space than you need. Resist it. Grow with your space.

If you can rent initially for one year, do that. Be certain you are happy with your location, hospitals, and the community of doctors in your area. Be certain you have selected the best geographic location for your practice and your family.

I remember trying to decide where I would set up my practice. I was in my final year of residency. This is a critical decision. It is not easy to move to another city after setting up a practice. Take your time and do your research. If you have a family, this should be a family decision, too. You will have to ask yourself many questions. Does your spouse work, and if so, where are his or her opportunities? Where will you send your children to school? How are the public and private school systems in the area? Are their churches or temples or mosques available to practice your faith? Is your extended family nearby?

I bought a large map and tacked it to my wall. This was before the era of Google Maps. I took a pin with a colored top and stuck it in the map wherever there was another dermatologist. I was trying to find a spot in South Florida with the fewest dermatologists. The cities with the most concentrated pins had the most dermatologists. I looked for an area within a city that had the fewest pins. I did not want to go where there were no dermatologists. Competition is a good thing. There is always room for another good physician.

Be a minimalist. Resist the fancy bathroom with a shower in your office. Get what you need to get your practice started. After renting for a short term, you will better know your needs for a more permanent solution. Buy rather than lease. Every physician I knew regretted not buying his or her space early in his or her career. Leasing prices escalate each year. It often becomes cost prohibitive. It may seem less expensive initially. It's not. It is easy to get a loan from the bank to buy space. Banks prefer loaning to physicians because the office space is "owner occupied." Assuming rates remain low, your mortgage payment may be less than your lease payment. The advantage to owning is that you will build valuable equity in the office. You may sell the office later or in retirement. As an owner, you will be the landlord and the tenant. I advise purchasing the office as a separate corporate entity such as an LLC (limited liability corporation). The LLC is the landlord and rents to your practice. Your practice corporation is the tenant. This protects you and your practice from the liabilities associated with owning the property.

THE OFFICE EQUIPMENT

Equipment requirements are generic to most office-based businesses. You will need a machine that can fax, copy, and scan. These systems come all as one or as separate, individual units. They are all inexpensive and can be found easily. You have many options to choose from.

I recommend that you accept credit cards. It is worth the small transaction fee. Frequently, patients claim that they "do not have their checkbook" to avoid paying at the time of service. We have trained our staff to respond by offering them the option of paying by credit card. Almost everyone has credit cards. The other advantage of accepting credit cards is that it reduces the likelihood of receiving bad checks. If you accept credit cards, you will need a credit card merchant and terminal to process the credit card payments. This can be done over the Internet or with a physical machine that swipes credit cards. There are many credit card merchants that you can bid out. It is a very competitive business, so let vendors compete over your business. Choose the vendor that offers the best service and lowest transaction rates.

You will need phones for the office. A phone system is expensive. It will provide functionality that other cheaper phones will not. You will need multiple lines, at least two at first. Lines should be set up to automatically roll over to the second line when the first one is busy. Patients should never receive a busy signal. Additionally, most phone systems come with conference calling capabilities, speakerphones, and intercom calling functions. As you grow, you may add additional lines. Initially, the second line may be used as a fax line. There are less expensive alternatives, such as Voice Over Internet Protocol (VOIP) phones, or virtual Web-based phone numbers with answering services. You can purchase a virtual Web-based fax service for relatively little expense. Performance issues still exist with an Internet-based telephone. Be cautious. This may cause you to lose patients if your phone systems do not work properly.

You business will require generic computer hardware. This includes desktops, monitors, and printers. Hardware is inexpensive and can be found easily. I would recommend PCs (personal computers) with a Windows operating system.

You will need to network your computers. Networking equipment is easy to find and is inexpensive. I would suggest deferring this to your IT (information technology) consultant. Your IT consultant will be your network expert. He or she should set up your computers, your network, and your Internet connectivity.

You will need varying selections of furniture for your office. This would be waiting room chairs and tables. You will need chairs for the exam rooms. You will need a desk for your office as well as work stations for the front office. There are many readily available sources for inexpensive chairs and furniture. I would suggest looking at used furniture stores and online sites first, as this may save you a lot of money.

You will need an exam table in each room. These may range from $500 to $20,000. The type of exam table you need will depend upon your specialty. In general, electric chairs are very expensive. I set up my practice by buying only used exam room furniture. I saved tens of thousands of dollars by doing this.

You will need medical supplies that are disposable, such as gauze, bandages, needles, alcohol, tongue depressors, and more, depending upon your specialty. These are commodity items and can be purchased from many large companies, such as PSS (Physician Sales and Services, Inc.). Additionally, your local medical society or national medical society may have formed "purchasing" groups. These groups obtain more competitive rates than purchasing individually in smaller volumes.

Table 14. A list of the minimum equipment categories you will need to start your practice:

1. Fax/copier/scanner

2. Credit card terminal/swiper/merchant vendor

3. Phones or phone system

4. Hardware and software

5. Networking equipment

6. Office furniture

7. Exam room furniture

THE PRACTICE MANAGEMENT CONSULTANT

When you first set up your practice, there may be a temptation to hire a practice management consultant. Although some may be great and helpful, many are often expensive and inefficient. I am not a big fan of practice management consultants, but many doctors are and have had excellent experiences with theirs. Reference sources like this book and the Internet make much of the information you need to set up your practice easily accessible.

The benefit of a good medical practice management consultant is that he or she can bring a new and unique perspective to analyzing your practice. A consultant may make business observations and suggestions that you would not otherwise think of. Be careful before you hire a practice management consultant. Ask him or her the questions found in Table 6 before you make your decision.

Table 15. Questions to ask a practice management consultant before hiring him or her:

1. How many years' experience in business do you have?

2. How many doctors' practices have you worked with?

3. What specialties have you worked with?

4. How many of those physician practices that your worked with do you continue to consult on and maintain?

5. Do you sell anything?

6. Do you work on any form of commission?

7. What are your fees? Hourly? Retainer?

8. What deliverables and reports do you guarantee you provide?

9. What if you are late on deliverables?

10. Do you provide free initial interviews?

PITFALLS TO AVOID

If you sign an agreement with a practice management consultant, make sure you can terminate your agreement at any time without penalty. Watch the "hold harmless" clauses so you do not indemnify the consultant for things that he or she does incorrectly. Make certain that there are penalties if he or she doesn't deliver on time. Be certain that you don't pay for work that is behind schedule, inadequate, or incomplete. Set up the agreement so that you pay only upon receiving deliverables. Define timeline milestones that you both agree are reasonable.

In summary, this chapter discussed issues surrounding picking an office location, leasing versus buying, and outfitting your office. Additionally, we touched upon the option of hiring a practice management consultant. We discussed the questions to ask before that decision is made. In the next chapter we cover the basics about advertising, marketing, and public relations. We cover the concept of lifetime value of a customer and customer acquisition costs.

MARKETING AND PUBLIC RELATIONS

The key to successful marketing and advertising is to understand the concept of "cost of acquisition" versus "lifetime value" of a patient. You should not spend a penny until you understand this concept. You must have a way to measure the effectiveness of your advertising. The "lifetime" value of a patient may be $300 (or more depending upon your specialty). That value is created through repeated visits over a patient's lifetime. This may represent several visits over the next few years. The cost of acquisition of that patient should always be less than the "lifetime" value of $300 (I will go into detail of this concept later).

Today it is much less expensive to market your practice than it was when I started fifteen years ago. That is entirely due to the Internet. In the early days, the Yellow Pages were the primary source of patients. Today I don't advertise at all in the Yellow Pages. The only advantage to placing any sort of advertising in the Yellow Pages is if it includes Internet exposure.

Marketing and advertising are two different ways to acquire patients. Advertising is spending money on ads to directly target your potential customer. Marketing is spending money to acquire customers through awareness that may include advertising but includes other ways, too.

Public relations (PR) is a form of marketing and not advertising. They are all important. I will discuss them in greater detail.

The most effective channel for marketing a practice is marketing to potential referring physicians. Market your practice by visiting their offices. Drop off your cards and shake their hands. Introduce yourself. Doctors enjoy that. They are used to it. A handshake goes a lot further than an introduction letter. Do both. Visit the hospital physicians' dining room for lunch daily. Send a thank-you note to doctors that refer patients, and include your business cards.

A marketing campaign will also include direct-to-patient marketing. Volunteer to give community lectures and participate at health care screening fairs. I still have patients that I acquired from my first health fair fifteen years ago. Every time we see each other, we reminisce about how we met at a health care fair. We laugh about how young I was. It's very rewarding.

Every marketing campaign must include an Internet strategy. This strategy includes promoting your Web site through a variety of initiatives. First and foremost, go to getlisted.org and register your practice with Google, Yahoo, and Bing.

Search engine optimization (SEO) means that your Web site is coded to enable search engines to recognize your site. Search engines use various sophisticated algorithms to recognize a Web site. If a search engine recognizes your site, then it will show up on the natural side of the search engine. The natural side is the left-hand side when using Google as an example. The right hand side of Google, for instance, is pay-per-click advertising. The complexity of coding your Web site is beyond my understanding, but there are many firms that can be hired to do this for you. I would recommend this.

Internet marketing strategy must include a social media component. Create a free Twitter account that links to your Web site. Create a free blog that links to your Web site. Create a Facebook page for your practice and link it to all your other social media sites.Use your Twitter and blog account to show that you are an expert in your field. When blogging or Tweeting, avoid the temptation to put in personal quotes, such as "in Las Vegas with friends about to hit the slots."

Table 16. Marketing campaigns

1. Referring physicians

2. Patients

3. Search engine optimization

4. Social media campaigns

5. Pay-per-click and pay-per-call campaigns

6. Direct mail

Advertising should be part of your Internet marketing campaign. Pay-per-click advertising and pay-per-call advertising are two options. Pay-per-click advertising means that you only get charged when someone clicks on your ad. You bid for the most common keywords that people use when searching for a doctor on the Internet. Most pay-per-click sites will help you optimize your advertisement by suggesting keywords that are relevant to your ad. For instance, if you are advertising a dermatology practice, then the sites will make "suggestions" for common keywords that people use when searching for dermatologists online. Your ad will show up on the right-hand side of Google when those keyword searches are used. However, your bid for keywords needs to be high enough that your ad shows up within the first one or two pages of the search. If you bid too low, your ad will show up behind many others. It won't be visible. You won't be charged until someone clicks on your ad. I caution that pay-per-click advertising can be inefficient and costly. You must understand this process or it will get very expensive. However, once you learn how to use it, you can make it work for your practice. You can set a daily limit on spending so that you can easily create a monthly budget. Keyword advertising is a science within itself and, for the purpose of this book, I will not go into detail. However, here are some good general tips:

(1) Use geography as a parameter for keyword advertising. The geography should be set so the ads only show up in an area that you think you would draw patients from. In my situation, I use thirty miles from my practice.

(2) Choose keywords that are relevant to your practice and not generic to all doctors. Be as specific as you can.

(3) Monitor your conversion rate so you can calculate your "cost of acquisition." How much does it cost to get a new patient? Calculate this by multiplying the amount spent divided by the number of new patients received in a given time period.

Pay-per-call advertising is different from pay-per-click advertising. Pay per call is newer and is available through certain Internet phone companies. This form of advertising only charges you when a potential customer calls an 800 number from your ad. The 800 number redirects to your office number. It is easy for the advertiser to monitor how many calls generate from the ad.

THE PUBLIC RELATIONS (PR) CAMPAIGN

Even as a doctor, a PR campaign can be valuable. If you want to be known as an expert in your field, you create a PR campaign to promote yourself through various media outlets: i.e., TV, radio, newspapers, and the Internet.

The expensive way to do this is hire a PR firm to represent you. It will charge you a monthly fee, plus it will charge you every time it gets you media exposure. PR firms are experts. They are often too expensive for a typical physician's budget.

The "poor man's" approach to PR is what I have done. There are companies like prnewswire.com that enable you to write your own press release. You can choose the media outlets that you want to distribute your release to. I have found this to be very effective and inexpensive. The service provides expertise. It will help you write your own press release. It is included in your fee. Your release will be distributed to journalists and editors over the news wires and on the Internet. This helps your Web site's optimization. It creates exposure and "buzz" about your practice.

When selecting a topic for a press release, make sure you are not writing an ad. Think in terms of what is newsworthy. Don't write a press release that claims that you are the best surgeon. That will not work. Don't write a press release that claims you offer a procedure at the best price. That is too generic and more of an ad. You need an angle. An example of an angle would be a human-interest story. An example of a human-interest story would be that you performed surgery without a fee on a child that was in need. People respond to physicians who do "pro bono" work.

Table 17. Ideas for a press release

1. Announce that you are the only physician providing a certain procedure in your area.

2. Announce that you have received a unique form of training.

3. Announce that your office has technology and services that are new to the area.

4. Announce that you are adding new state-of-the-art equipment that no other physician has in the area.

5. Show how you are treating patients without charge for certain disorders.

In this chapter we discussed the difference between advertising and public relations. We provided ideas for Internet marketing and press releases. We discussed the importance of understanding cost of acquisition and lifetime value of a customer before creating a marketing budget.

CONCLUSION

There is a deficiency in the curriculum of medical school and residency programs. It is in the business of medicine. The emphasis, understandably, is on the clinical practice of medicine. The reality is that business plays such a prominent role in every doctor's postresidency career that this deficiency is significant. Medical students should receive business education during medical school and residency. There are no courses on this subject. There are no textbooks required for medical students on business. Yet every doctor is confronted with business issues daily.

Hopefully, the first section of this book provided you with the foundations needed to enter into private practice. The topics I covered are the building blocks necessary to help doctors lay the groundwork for entering medical practice. They are business essentials. Many of these issues I learned after making mistakes on my own. A book like this was not available when I completed my residency. There are resources for doctors such as the American Medical Association Web site. However, they still assume a basic understanding of business. They do not educate doctors on business fundamentals. They do not educate physicians on reading a balance sheet or understanding the nuances between a subchapter C and a subchapter S corporation. They do not cover negotiating lines of credit, for example. The issues covered in the first part of this book are everyday business issues. They are relevant. They are my experiences, mistakes and successes. I am sharing them with you. And, they will help you from the moment you decide you want to go into private practice.

Medicine has given me many options. As a resident, I struggled with the decision between an academic career and a career in private practice. I felt that I was a "sellout" for not staying in academics. After fifteen years, nothing could be further from the truth. I have enjoyed all of it. The business aspect of medicine is exciting. The patient relationships are rewarding. The smartest move I made was going out on my own and establishing a solo practice. Most doctors would consider this too risky today. I don't. When I did it, everyone was afraid that managed care would ruin the profession forever. The naysayers in the eighties would have told you to avoid private practice because of HMOs (health maintenance organizations) and PPOs (preferred provider organizations). Although physician income was reduced, opportunities still remained for entrepreneurial physicians. I took the risk. I suggest you do the same.

Go into private practice. You will not regret it. You will have the creative freedom to shape the practice into a business. The business will reflect your own interests and personality. This is rewarding. You will form exciting and long-lasting relationships with dedicated employees. This is enduring. You will see families grow up and experience life's pains and joys with them. This is heartwarming. You will never forget the challenges you encountered and overcame in creating a successful practice. This book prepares you for them. This is a promise.

PART II:

For all physician entrepreneurs

The entrepreneurial bug bit me a few years into my practice. The business was managing itself. I had the time to recognize other opportunities within my practice. I wanted to parlay those ideas into another business or, at a minimum, create additional revenue streams for the practice.

This section of the book details my experience in creating several new businesses. Their genesis arose from my practice experiences. It is hard for a doctor to create a new business entity separate from the practice. It is even harder to run both a practice and an unrelated business venture simultaneously. More often than not, both suffer. However, many doctors try. I want to pass on my experiences to you so that you may learn from them.

I am a physician entrepreneur. If you are reading this book, then you are, too. Physician entrepreneurs are creative doctors who are excited by the challenge of founding a new business. Doctors receive no formal training in business or the entrepreneurial process. A physician entrepreneur is entering unchartered waters and flying blind. The process is highly complex, sophisticated, and challenging. Unlike the low risk and consistent financial returns that result from creating a solo medical practice, being an entrepreneur is a high-risk, high-return scenario. It can be costly financially and emotionally. The financial returns may be great, but the risks are greater.

I am excited to share with you my adventures. These are the adventures of a serial physician entrepreneur. The last fifteen years have been a roller-coaster ride for me. I hope to capture this for you. The goal of this section is to teach you about the following entrepreneurial topics through sharing my real-life examples with you.

1. The genesis of a new business idea.
2. Understanding a balance sheet and your capital needs in a start-up company.
3. The nuances of raising capital.
4. Expertise in the field you are starting the new venture in.
5. The time commitment of a start-up.
6. Management team and staff.
7. Advisory boards.
8. Contracts and leases.
9. When things go bad...really bad...don't panic, and remember your poker face.

AN IDEA AND A DREAM

It started in 1996. Every time I picked up *Business 2.0* magazine, the cover had a story about another twentysomething that had raised tens of millions of dollars to fund a ridiculous idea. It was the "dotcom" days, and there were many paper millionaires. I wasn't one of them.

I remember the moment clearly. It was the first time I decided to do something unrelated to my practice. I was in my home office. My medical practice was doing well and on autopilot. I had recently added over-the-counter dispensing to my practice. We started dispensing a few new skin-care products called cosmeceuticals. This was an additional passive revenue source for my practice. Passive revenue was incremental revenue that resulted from not actively seeing patients, i.e., passive. Cosmeceuticals were a niche industry that was just starting to take off. They were neither pharmaceuticals nor cosmetics. They did not need a prescription, as they were not drugs. They worked to make the appearance of the skin better. Cosmeceuticals were quickly growing to become a billion-dollar industry. Before 1996, you had to visit a dermatologist or plastic surgeon's office to buy cosmeceuticals. That was the opportunity. I realized that it was ridiculous to force a patient to come to the office to purchase over-the-counter, nonprescription skin care creams. In 1996 I decided to sell the products

I was selling in my office online. At that time no one did that. Today hundreds, if not thousands, do that.

I incorporated my idea and came up with the name Skinstore.com. I had no technology experience, so I asked a college buddy who had a Web design company to create a Web site for me. The key to the business was ease. The products I sold were products I already inventoried for my office. I wrote every page of content on the site and included an education center. The online education center was written for people to click to learn about their skin conditions. Twelve years ago, that was a novel idea. I tested the Web site to see if people would actually buy products from Skinstore.com. My college buddy also was an expert with online advertising. Between the copy I wrote and the keyword advertising he placed, orders started coming in. Initially I filled the orders using plain boxes in my office. However, quickly the orders outgrew my capacity to both fill the orders and maintain running of my medical practice. At this point, I needed help.

Skinstore.com was disruptive. It created problems for the manufacturer, distributor, and the retailer. The Internet was creating this dilemma for many industries. All of a sudden, a distributor was being replaced by a Web site. The wholesalers did not know what to do. In Skinstore's scenario specifically, the manufacturers and wholesalers did not want me to sell online. They wanted to protect their physician customers that were dispensing in their office. Skinstore was not well received initially. I knew that and wasn't sure how to handle it at first.

My first challenge was to be certain that the manufacturers continued to sell the product wholesale to my dermatology practice. I needed that product to sell online through Skinstore. Skinstore could not buy the product directly.

I intentionally kept my name off the Skinstore Web site. The manufacturers could not easily find out where Skinstore was getting its product. Skinstore received several "cease and desist" letters. The letters threatened legal action if I did not stop selling unauthorized products through the Skinstore Web site. I ignored them. I knew that ultimately I was helping the manufacturer by selling its product. The manufacturer just didn't realize how big this could be.

The big breakthrough for Skinstore came when I purchased a full-page advertisement in a major national magazine. I was able to find manufacturers to fund the cost of the ad. Skinstore did not threaten them. They embraced the new channel since they were already in retail. I leveraged my relationship with these two companies from my dermatology practice. I negotiated a deal to advertise two separate products: Dermablend and Mederma. Both products benefitted from the ad. Skinstore's revenue and sales took off. I knew I had a business.

In order to grow the company, we needed to invest significant dollars into it. I decided to raise outside capital from friends and family. I wrote a business plan. Until that time, my role had been president and chief executive officer of Skinstore. I decided to keep my practice going and hired a CEO to replace me.

Twelve months had passed. B2C (business direct to consumer model) companies were falling out of favor with institutional investors. In response, we created another distribution model for our company. It was a B2B (business to business model). B2B companies were highly sought after. We renamed the company. The model was to provide dermatologists and plastic surgeons with Web sites, products, information, education, and tools to make their practices more efficient. This business was received very well. We created an outstanding advisory board with nationally recognized thought leaders. It included many Harvard professors. We raised approximately $2.5 million at a valuation of $6 million. Once you have raised capital, you have gone from a simple company with one owner to a more complex one with many owners.

Everyone has an idea. Everyone has a business that he or she knows will work. Very few people actually execute on their ideas. It is a huge leap to go from a good idea to creating a business. Most people underestimate the task. Most people are unprepared for the time demands and competition. If you have a dream to create a business, go for it. Be prepared. The endeavor comes at a cost. Initially, your "capital" investment will be your energy and free time. This investment is not recoverable. As you get further along, the investment will become real money, either from you or from investors. If you believe in your idea, do not be derailed by naysayers. Stay committed. You will hit resistance at every turn. Enjoy it. Treasure the experience. It is much different than seeing patients every day.

The next section will help you understand the capital demands of a new company. This is the critical first step before raising money. Raising money is critical to every entrepreneurial venture. It is the lifeline of the company. Raise too much and you will dilute your ownership interest. Raise too little money and you will not be able to fund the company.

UNDERSTANDING FINANCIAL STATEMENTS, INTELLECTUAL PROPERTY, AND RAISING CAPITAL

In this section we will cover how much money you really need to start a business. We will teach you how to read a balance sheet. We will help you understand the realities of capital costs. Then, we will discuss how you raise the capital to meet your needs.

Do not start any business unless you have raised or set aside enough money to cover expenses and payroll for a minimum of three years. This is the single biggest mistake most, if not all, entrepreneurs make. The capital demands of the business are underappreciated. And, this is the reason that 90 percent of businesses fail within the first three years.

If you do not have at least three years of expenses (including your salary and payroll) in the form of liquid capital set aside, you are doomed to fail even before you start. You will be forced to focus much of your time and efforts on raising additional money. You won't be able to be focus on the critical aspects of growing and operating the business. The challenge is projecting how much capital will be "burned" or spent during the first three years of your business. You must create honest and objective cash flow projections.

Assume the following for the purposes of creating realistic cash flow projections: you will have no revenue for two years, expenses will be 2.5 times your projections, and you will not get your product to market on time. There are always many complicated and unpredictable variables that cause these problems. You should expect that.

"Burn rate" is a term that refers to how much money you will spend per month keeping the company alive. It derives from your original projected P&L (profit and loss) statement and cash flow projections. Unforeseen variables will arise and force you to revise your cash flow estimates. Revisions impact your burn rate and affect the amount of cash remaining for continued operations. Many of these changes are due to factors beyond your control, such as regulatory, manufacturing, and parts issues, for example. Most entrepreneurs will underestimate true costs and incur unexpected problems. These problems will eat up your funding sooner than planned.

Every entrepreneur should know how to read and understand a financial statement. The financials include the P&L or income statement, cash flow statement and balance sheet.

A financial statement that measures the financial performance of a company over a specific accounting period is known as the P&L statement or income statement or statement of revenue and expense. This statement summarizes how a company incurs revenues and expenses through operating and nonoperating activities. Operating activities are a direct result of regular business operations. An example would be selling hamburgers at Burger King. Nonoperating activities that result in income or expenses would be those not related to regular business. An example of this would be selling land, equipment, or a building owned by the business.

In its simplest form, a balance sheet is a numerical representation of what a business owns and what a business owes. The difference between these numbers is the "paper" value of the company. The balance sheet is a snapshot of the company's health at any given time. It is based on the formula that assets equal liabilities plus shareholder equity. Assets are what a company uses to operate. Liabilities and shareholder equity support the assets. Shareholder equity is the amount of money initially invested in the company, plus retained earnings. Retained earnings are the net earnings retained fiscally by the company and not paid out as dividends. These earnings are used to reinvest in the company. Reinvestment may be in the form of equipment or research and development. Retained earnings are part of the shareholders' equity. They are calculated by adding net income to initial retained earnings and subtracting dividends paid to shareholders. Thus, earnings from the income statement that are reinvested in the company become booked as retained earnings on the balance sheet.

There are two different types of assets: current and noncurrent. Current assets include cash, accounts receivable, and inventory. Noncurrent assets include tangible assets and nontangible assets. Tangible assets include equipment, computers, land, and buildings. Intangible assets include goodwill, patents, intellectual property, and copyrights. Depreciation is deducted from the value of all assets. Depreciation represents the economic cost of the asset over the asset's useful lifetime.

In order for a balance sheet to balance out, the assets must equal the liabilities plus shareholder equity. The information provided in the balance sheet provides a picture of the financial strength of a company. Analysis includes financial ratios, such as working capital and debt-to-equity ratio. Working capital equals current assets minus current liabilities. Positive working capital means a company can meet its current short-term liabilities, while the converse is true for negative working capital. Debt-to-equity ratios can be calculated by dividing debt by shareholder equity. A high debt-to-equity ratio implies that a company has been aggressive in financing its growth through debt. The expense of this debt may impact the bottom line and create volatility for the company.

The cash flow statement provides information on the cash inflows and outflows of the company. Cash may inflow from a variety of sources, such as revenue or external investors. Cash may outflow for a variety of reasons, such as operations and investments made by the company. The cash flow statement is different from the income statement. It provides a better snapshot of the actual cash on hand by the company at a given time. Sometimes the income statement will reflect booked income on sales for cash not yet received. It is important to understand this difference so that cash flow and burn rates can be managed.

In order to create these cash flow and P&L projections, you must detail your expected expenses. Expenses impact your funding requirements. A P&L statement will include all the expenses that you expect to have each year.

The following are examples of the initial expenses you should expect before you have sold even one product.

Incorporating your business will be the first expense that you have. You will need to incorporate as an LLC (limited liability corporation), subchapter S corporation, or subchapter C corporation. There are advantages and disadvantages for each type of corporation. You should consult an accountant before making an election. (I have already discussed this in great detail in Part 1 of this book and will cover it only in generalities here).

In general, LLCs and S corporations afford personal liability protection and allow pass-through of losses to personal income. The C corporation is structured to allow for a greater numbers of shareholders. It allows for health care benefits to be expensed by the corporation. It poses a risk of double taxation. Double taxation means that both the corporation and the individual owner pay income taxes.

In a limited liability corporation (LLC), the corporate entity generally protects shareholders and directors from the debts and obligations of the company. In contrast, in a partnership or sole proprietorship, the owner's personal assets are at risk and may be used to pay business debts.

One difference between a subchapter S corporation and an LLC is that corporations can issue stock while an LLC issues membership certificates instead of stock. The sale of stock is the easiest way to attract outside investors.

Some of the advantages of a subchapter S corporation over a subchapter C corporation:

1. avoidance of double taxation;
2. taxes may be less on sale of business if S corporation;
3. pass-through of income and losses to the individual owner's return.

Each corporation type has specific requirements that must be met in order to make that election. The requirements for a subchapter S corporation are:

1. each S corporation shareholder must be a U.S. citizen or resident;
2. the S corporation can never have more than seventy-five shareholders;
3. S corporation profits or losses must be allocated in direct proportion to ownership interests;

4. the corporation may not deduct the cost of fringe benefits provided to employee-shareholders that own more than 2 percent of the corporation.

I recommend that you incorporate any new, separate business entity (i.e., separate from your medical practice) in the state of Delaware. A Delaware corporation has the most favorable tax considerations. Here is a list of the benefits of incorporating in Delaware:

1. Delaware has no personal property tax, intangible property tax, or sales tax levied against Delaware corporations.
2. Delaware corporations do not pay state income tax.
3. Delaware corporations owned by nonresidents are not subject to any Delaware taxes.
4. Incorporating in Delaware involves no minimum capital requirement, while many other states require at least $1,000 in capital. Delaware corporations can be formed at a low cost.
5. Incorporating in Delaware is an easy process. The Delaware Corporation Department has developed a customer-friendly and easy way for corporations to incorporate in Delaware.
6. One person can be the only officer, director, and shareholder for Delaware corporations.
7. No additional people are required to fill the director or officer positions of Delaware corporations.
8. Delaware corporations pay low incorporation costs when incorporating in Delaware.
9. Delaware corporations can be formed without visiting Delaware.
10. Meetings of Delaware corporations can be held anywhere and need not be in Delaware.

11. Delaware corporations pay an annual franchise tax that is amongst the lowest in the nation.
12. Many companies that may acquire you in the future prefer Delaware corporations.

STAT CONSULT FROM JOHN IGOE, A CORPORATE ATTORNEY

S Corporation vs. LLC: The owners of an S corporation must be U.S. individual resident taxpayers; with minor exceptions, trusts and corporations are not permitted to hold stock in S corporations. LLCs have grown in popularity because they provide the same type of flow-through or single-tax treatment as S corporations, with no limit on the number or nature of members.

Incorporating in Delaware is a common approach, especially if you anticipate that your company will need to raise venture capital. Most public companies are incorporated in Delaware because the laws generally favor corporations (vs. shareholder rights) and the volume of case law in Delaware has provided guidelines and blueprints for corporations and lawyers to follow. Delaware has taken advantage of this by charging annual franchise fees based on authorized capital stock. This can be very costly. However, there is a formula available tied to asset values for reducing the tax for smaller companies.

Wherever you incorporate, the founders should invest a reasonable amount of initial capital. The company will need the money. The founders should invest something of value for their stock. Also, without some level of capital, this could be a factor enabling creditors to pierce the corporate veil and establish personal liability of the principals for debts of the company.

Intellectual property expenses need to be accounted for in your initial projections. Intellectual property is the creative property associated with your business. It can be tangible, or it may be intangible and conceptual. Intellectual property includes logos, trademarks, patents, designs, concepts, plans, Web sites, and technologies, or even business ideas written on scraps of napkins at the dinner table.

Intellectual property includes patents. The process of applying for a patent is expensive. The process of protecting and defending the patent is exorbitant. Only in certain businesses and limited scenarios are patents critical to the success of a start-up. There are many companies that have spent hundreds of thousands of dollars to create patents for their companies before they launch. I would advise against paying for patents unless your business model is entirely dependent upon patent protection. If so, be prepared to spend thousands of dollars defending your patent against large corporations that notice your success.

One approach I have used with patents is what I call the "poor man's" option to patents. I have done this with my companies. Apply for "patent pending" status. This is less expensive, and the legal work is much less. You will need to fill out a full patent application within two years of your patent pending status. Patent pending will protect your idea, put you in line with the patent office, and may help you raise capital. The patent pending application should cost anywhere between $5,000 and $10,000 with an IP (intellectual property) attorney. After the patent pending status period is over, you must file a complete patent application. Two years will have passed and you may have raised significant dollars by that time.

Trademarks and copyrights are useful. They can be done very inexpensively. I filed all my own trademarks online at uspto.gov. The cost to file is under $500. Attorneys will do exactly the same thing for you, but for a fee. I recommend doing this without an attorney. Other creative costs include logo development and tagline development.

Naming the company and registering the Web domain are critical. Be certain the domain name is available before naming the company. It is not unusual to name a company and find out later that the domain name is not available. Purchase the domain name for a minimum of three years from a reliable provider like GoDaddy or Network Solutions. I would suggest buying the .com, .net, and .tel suffixes for the domain name that you have chosen.

STAT CONSULT FROM HOWARD M. GITTEN, AN INTELLECTUAL PROPERTY ATTORNEY

1. INTELLECTUAL PROPERTY: THE REAL VALUE OF THE COMPANY

Every entrepreneur thinks he or she has a competitive advantage. If you don't think you have a competitive advantage, go back to your day job, because if you do not perceive a differentiating value add in your proposition, then you are doomed to become a commodity. However, if you have a better mousetrap, a better way of selling that mousetrap, or a more cost-efficient way of building that mousetrap, then you can compete in the marketplace. Traditionally, businesses have thought of their physical assets, such as land, buildings, equipment, even the products themselves, as their most valuable assets. However, a company's intellectual assets, those things which provide for a competitive advantage, i.e., intellectual property, may in fact be your most valuable assets.

Intellectual property has value to customers in the perceived value of your product, to potential strategic partners in the rights that you may convey, and to investors because of the value intellectual property brings a company, especially an early stage company.

Intellectual property can be protected in four ways. There are patents, trademarks, copyrights, and trade secrets. Each will be discussed below.

II. A PATENT

What Is It?

A patent is a right granted by the federal government which protects a concept. It is protection for the idea itself. It may protect that process for manufacture (curing rubber tires, therapies), the manner in which software controls a computer to perform a function (a search engine), devices (a cell phone, the tire itself), compositions of material (pharmaceuticals, new resins, rubbers), or any new and useful improvement thereof. The special type of patent known as a design patent protects the ornamental design for manufactured products, such as a watch face or the shape of a toy (Star Trek Enterprise). Lastly, plant patents may be obtained for new varieties of plants that can be reproduced asexually.

Somewhat counterintuitively, a patent does not grant you the right to make your device. Rather, it is a grant from the federal government conferring the right to exclude others from making, selling, or using an invention. In other words, it gives you the right to stop others.

How Do I Get Mine?

Patents are not just granted to anyone with an idea. First, you must prove that the idea is useful; in other words, it must have utility. Someone trying to patent a law of nature, such as gravity, or a math theorem, or an impossibility such as a perpetual motion machine, will not pass the utility test. Most things are useful. However, once you prove that a concept is useful, you must prove to the government that your concept is novel. It must be different from what has come before; after all, you are claiming you really have an invention. Lastly, even if it is new, it must be unobvious to a person of ordinary skill in the art. If your new product is a car, then being the first person to paint the car purple is novel. However, it would be obvious, because we knew about the color purple, and we knew how to paint cars, so painting the first purple car is a mere design choice and obvious. However, if you are the first person to put a turbo charger in an engine to get more power, then this is not quite as obvious.

As shown above, anything under the sun with the exception of mathematical formulas and laws of nature can theoretically be patented. However, the process is not a rubber stamp. So how do you get your patent?

First, once you have your concept, you write a patent application, often with the help of a patent attorney. A patent application has three basic parts. The first section explains what is wrong with the world, i.e., what is the need for your idea. The second section is a detailed disclosure of what you are doing, explained well enough so that anybody reading your patent would know how to do it.

The tradeoff for the government monopoly is teaching the world your invention. Last is the claims section, which sets out in language what you claim as your idea.

Once completed, the application is then filed with the government. There are literally buildings full of patent examiners whose job is to make sure that your concept is useful, novel, and not obvious. The examiners look at public information which was known prior to your conception of your invention. This is a back-and-forth process, and once you prove to the examiner that in fact your concept has utility and is new and unobvious, the government issues you a patent.

What Good Is It?

The patent is a monopoly to prevent others from making, using, selling, or importing your concept. It is a limited monopoly in that it normally lasts for twenty years from the filing date of your application, and only extends to the idea described in the claims.

Once your patent has been granted, where is the value? First, because it is a right to prevent others from using your idea, you can create a monopoly within your niche by refusing to give others the right to use your idea. On the other hand, you can monetize your concept by allowing others to use your idea. However, they must pay you for that use. This is the royalty rate for the license to use your concept.

When someone uses your idea without authorization, that is known as patent infringement. You must look to the claims and determine whether or not the invention defined in the patent claims covers the competing device.

If so, then you can demand a royalty payment or sue to stop them from making, using, or selling your invention.

Many times, you may need the permission of others to launch your product. If you as an inventor obtained a patent for a new kind of medical device and that medical device infringes on a prior patent owned by Baxter, then you still have no right to make, use, or sell your medical device. To do so, you will need to obtain permission from Baxter. Baxter may refuse the permission, or ask that a royalty be paid for the rights to infringe on its patent.

We should note that patent litigation is the sport of kings. A typical patent infringement case costs each side at least $1 million to litigate all the way through to trial. However, because it is so expensive, the threat of litigation is an effective tool for getting a competitor to stop making, using, or selling your product, or to take a license.

TRADEMARKS (this section on trademarks was also covered in Part I of this book)

What Are They?

Trademarks protect the goodwill of your company. They in effect identify your company as the source of certain goods of a certain quality. A trademark is any word, name, symbol, or device used to identify the source or origin of products or services and to distinguish those products or services from others. When you hear McDonald's, it has a different connotation in your mind than Burger King, even for very similar products. You as a consumer know what to expect when you eat at McDonald's. Now think how confusing it would be and how upset McDonalds would be if Burger King changed the name of its famous burger to the McWhopper.

Everyone knows that words such as Sprite soda, Corvette convertible, and Google searches are valid and appropriate use of trademarks. It is also well known that numbers and letters have become very famous trademarks, such as BMW, 3M, and 1-800-FLOWERS as a source of goods and services; and, lastly, designs and logos also have great power as trademarks. Think of the Nike swoosh, Adidas stripes, Starbucks' mermaid; all very strong trademarks in the mind of the consumer.

However, less conventional identifiers can also be used as trademarks. For example, sounds such as the roar of the MGM lion, the opening notes of Microsoft software, and even an attempt to trademark the Harley- Davidson engine sound. Fragrances such as stationery treated with a special fragrance can be trademarks. Shapes such as the unique shape of the Apple iPod or Lego building blocks have been given trademark protection. Colors such as the brown for UPS, Nexium's purple pill, and the distinctive pink, blue, and yellow artificial sweetener packets have all been used to establish brand awareness. I am sure that each of you, when reading this, has already identified the owners of the respective artificial sweetener colors; that is the ultimate test as to whether something has become a trademark. Lastly, the overall look, the trade dress, has been given trademark protection. For example, a distinctive décor and layout for most franchise restaurants, such as Hooters' orange and white uniforms and wooden décor or Chipotle's accent colors, metal, and wood, would be given trademark protection.

The government, in effect, is giving you a monopoly over a word and its use in commerce. So, like patents, there are certain hurdles which must be overcome in order to establish the strength and validity of your trademark. Words may be generic, descriptive, suggestive, or fanciful. Where your proposed trademark lies on that spectrum will govern the strength of its use as a trademark. By way of example, if you are a farmer and you wish to brand your new red, shiny fruit APPLE, the government will not grant you trademark rights, because apple is generic for the red, shiny fruit. What would other farmers call their red, shiny fruit?

Similarly, if you are a baker and you wish to trademark your cakes and cookies which taste like the red, shiny fruit, whether they include the red, shiny fruit or artificial ingredients, as APPLE cookies, you will not be allowed to enforce monopoly rights in that brand either. Such use is descriptive. How would other bakeries describe their apple-flavored products? Therefore, descriptive marks are, for the most part, not enforceable.

However, if you are manufacturing a perfume which smells sweet or fruity and wish to brand that perfume APPLE perfume, then the word is only suggestive of a characteristic of the product, and you will most likely be entitled to trademark protection. Better yet, if you are starting a computer company and name your product line APPLE, then this is fanciful and a strong mark.

However, words can change their status, and the spectrum discussed above is only a general yardstick. History is littered with examples of marks across the spectrum, including famous marks which have become generic. Generic marks such as "aspirin" and "thermos" both began as fanciful marks; Movie Channel or Healthy Choice may be considered descriptive bordering on suggestive marks.

Suggestive marks are marks such as Priceline.com, and fanciful marks are marks like Kodak and Windows.

There are other rules as to which types of marks are not acceptable for protection even if fanciful. Immoral or scandalous matter, such as curse words, will most likely not be granted trademark protection. Deceptive matter such as "Fresh Florida Oranges" for oranges grown in California, or anywhere other than Florida, will not be granted protection. Lastly, surnames such as Anderson or Smith or famous names such as Johnny Carson can't be trademarked unless you are that person or the person is fictitious.

How Do I Get Mine?

Unlike a patent, which must be issued by the government, you do not need the government to obtain a trademark right. There are registered trademarks, those which have ® as an indicator of government issuance, and common law trademarks indicated by ™. Both are valid marks. The government grants the trademark rights in the registered ® trademark. Common law trademark (TM) rights develop over time with use in commerce until they become so famous that they have meaning in the general public as being from a single source.

The process for obtaining a trademark always begins with selecting an appropriate mark; one that is not scandalous, deceptive, descriptive, or generic. Then a trademark search should be performed to make sure that the mark is free for use and that you are not infringing the rights of others. This can be done by consulting an attorney, or at least preliminarily conducting an Internet word search or a search at USPTO.gov, where all pending and currently registered trademarks can be searched. Once you have cleared the mark, the rights in the trademark are created either through extensive commercial use, including advertising and promotion of the brand embodied by the trademark, or by filing with the government for registration.

Similar to the patent process, the trademark registration process begins with an application in which you identify the name or any special artwork associated with the word, such as a logo and a description of the goods and services being provided under that brand. Again, there are buildings full of examiners who determine first whether the word is appropriate to be a trademark and then make sure that it does not cause a likelihood of confusion with any other pending or registered mark (registrations of similar words for similar goods). It should be noted that as part of the government process, the government only screens marks in its system when determining a likelihood of confusion. However, it may look outside of the U.S. Patent and Trademark Office to determine whether or not a mark is deceptive, profane, generic, or descriptive.

What Good Are They?

Once trademark rights are established, they are rights to prevent others from using words in a manner which is confusingly similar to the way in which you use your trademark. Trademark infringement occurs when there is a likelihood of confusion between someone else's uses of a word (not necessarily the identical word) in a confusing manner. At the heart of the test is (1) a determination of how close in sound and connotation to the actual trademarks are; (2) how close the goods associated with each word are; (3) what the overlap is in the channels of trade for the goods covered by the competing trademarks; and (4) how smart are the customers for the respective goods. By way of example, there is a very small likelihood of confusion between Cadillac automobiles and Cadillac dog food. However, if Coors started selling Coke beer, then Coca Cola, the soda company, would most likely be suing the beer company. Like patents, these rights can be used to stop others from infringing your trademarks, or as a way to license others to use your brand with similar or even different goods.

IV. COPYRIGHTS

What Are They?

Copyrights protect the form of expression and, more particularly, the form of expression fixed in a tangible medium. They don't protect the idea, the goods, the service, the goodwill, or even the oral presentation, although copyrighted materials can add to the value of all those things.

Copyright can be a very powerful right that grants the author, and any subsequent owner of a work, the legal rights to determine how that work is used in order to obtain the economic benefits from the work. Ironically, although copyrights are always considered to protect art, the work does not have to have artistic merit to be eligible for copyright protection. As a result, such things as operating manuals, computer software, and sales brochures are all eligible for copyright protection.

Everyone knows that literary works, such as magazine articles, books, plays, and musical compositions, are protectable by copyright. Computer software, pictorial, graphic, and even sculptural works, such as paintings, the artwork for a logo, and 3D models, are also protected by copyright; so are dramatic works. Even pantomimes and choreographic works, such as dance routines, can avail themselves of copyright protection when provided in a fixed medium.

Once again, the dance performance, if ad-libbed, cannot avail itself of such protection. So, how would you, as an author, protect your sighting of Elvis? Well, as you should have surmised by now, copyright law does not protect sightings or even the idea of selling photographs of Elvis. However, copyright law will protect your photo, painting, sound recording, or any other depiction of your Elvis sighting. No one can lawfully use your photo of your sighting, although someone else may copyright his or her own photo of his or her own sighting. Copyright law protects the original photograph, even the story you may write, but not the subject of the photograph. Therefore, although copyright is very effective for preventing others from copying your source code or your product documentation, it does not prevent others from independently creating their own source code which may be very similar, even identical to what you have created.

How Do I Get Mine?

Technically, it is not necessary to register the work with the United States Copyright Office. However, to enhance copyright protection, if possible, you should put copyright notice in the form of the copyright symbol ©, name of copyright owner, and year of first publication on each copy of the work. For example, my notice for this chapter, if standing alone, would be © Howard M. Gitten 2010. This puts the world on notice that this is a copyrighted work. Like trademarks, there are common law copyrights and registered copyrights. By registering your new work in the United States Copyright Office, further protection can be obtained in the United States, such as the ability to bring lawsuits to enforce your copyright.

What Good Is It?

As a copyright owner, you can prevent others from making, and in some cases even distributing, copies of your work. Copyright infringement occurs when one work is an exact copy or shows substantial similarity to the original work, and actual copying occurred. To prove infringement, you will be required to show that the alleged infringer had prior access to your copyrighted work and that the work is substantially similar to yours, i.e., some copying occurred. By way of example, the illegal downloading of music is copyright infringement; even sampling (taking small portions of your Web site art) can be infringement. There is no need to copy the copyrighted work in its entirety. The penalties for copyright infringement are quite draconian. Like trademarks and patents, you can stop others from making use of your copyrighted material and sue them for a penalty of up to $250,000 per copy.

Again, it should be noted that because copyrights give you, as the author or the copyright owner, the right to stop the use by others, copyrights lend themselves to commercialization. They can be licensed, sold, or used to keep others out of your competitive niche.

V. TRADE SECRETS

What Are They?

So far, each of the rights we have discussed utilizes a formalized process which may, if desired, be blessed by the government to grant certain rights. Trade secrets arise and are maintained solely by the acts of the person asserting the trade secret. A trade secret is any formula, pattern, physical device, idea, process, or other information that provides the owner of that information with a competitive advantage in the marketplace. This may include marketing plans, product formulas, financial forecasts, employee rosters, customer lists, logs of sales calls, and similar types of proprietary information. This can be very valuable. By way of example, Coca-Cola is a company founded on a secret formula, as is Kentucky Fried Chicken. Although their trademarks are extremely valuable these days, that branding was in part based on advertisement of their competitive niche, which in truth was a flavor differentiator resulting from a trade secret formula.

So what qualifies for a trade secret? In general, information that is known to the public or that competitors can discover through legal means doesn't qualify for trade secret protection. Once you launch your product, if it can be immediately reverse-engineered, then that product should be patented if possible because it would not qualify for trade secret protection. The strongest case for trade secret protection is information that has the following characteristics:

(a) The information is valuable and provides the company a competitive advantage.

(b) It is not known outside the company.

(c) Even inside the company, it is known on a need-to-know basis.

(d) It cannot be easily duplicated, reverse-engineered, or discovered.

(e) The information is safeguarded by stringent efforts to keep the secret.

If your information has these characteristics, then it lends itself to being protected by trade secret.

How Do I Get Mine?

There is no registration of a trade secret. No government agency grants the right. There is only maintenance of what you believe may be a trade secret. Simple steps and continuous effort maintain the value of the trade secret. Steps may include the clear differentiation between public areas and private areas at your facility, and the restriction of access not only to the private areas, but even within the private areas, such as further restriction of access to select personnel. Documents which are disseminated within the private areas should be labeled "confidential" to remind people of the duty of care required. Don't leave trade secret information where it can be easily seen, such as on a white board. Maintain log books for visitors to determine whether anyone may have access to your trade secret (to provide theft of the trade secret). Always use confidentiality and nondisclosure agreements when disclosing trade secrets to necessary individuals such as vendors, outsource manufacturers, even potential strategic partners. However, even under the umbrella of nondisclosure agreements, the scope of disclosure in both content and personnel should be on a need-to-know basis. These agreements are not a license to tell every secret under the sun.

For example, where a software development is the core of your value ad, password protection of the source code and extremely limited printed copies are ways to restrict access. Even then, the password should only be given on a need-to-know basis. Printed copies of the source code should be kept in limited-access cabinets and marked "Confidential" on their face.

What Good Are They?

There are shortcomings to relying on trade secret protections. First, once you decide to go the trade secret route, it is mutually exclusive to patent protection because patents are public documents. Secondly, once a competitor legitimately figures out your trade secret through his or her own legitimate efforts, a trade secret is not enforceable against that party. If you stumble upon the formula for making Coke soda in your own lab, Coke cannot stop you from competing. Thirdly, maintaining a trade secret requires effort and vigilance, which take time and effort. However, trade secrets can last theoretically forever. Again, Coke has been living off a trade secret for over a century.

In order to enforce a trade secret, much like copyright protection, the owner of the trade secret must demonstrate that the thief had access to the trade secret and had utilized the trade secret without authorization or permission (rather than reverse engineering), and, lastly, that steps were taken to preserve the secrecy of the trade secret by the trade secret owner. Otherwise, the trade secret may be considered to be part of the public domain. If theft of trade secret is proven, you can get an injunction to stop your competitors from using your trade secret as well as collect money based on their use of your trade secret.

IV. CONCLUSION

Hopefully, as can be seen by this brief discussion, intellectual property is valuable. It includes a bundle of rights with *overlapping protections. However, it requires effort and resources to establish and maintain ownership rights through registration, internal controls, and effective contracts (see attached chart). However, if done successfully, intellectual property assets can be commercially leveraged through business relationships, protecting a niche monopoly, or actually collecting royalties for their use. Therefore, time and effort should be put into determining which, if any, intellectual property rights should be established at the very outset of your venture.*

STATCCONSULT FROM JOHN IGOE, A CORPORATE ATTORNEY

I agree 100% with Dr. Hacker's advice to secure your domain name before incorporating your company. There are actually "swindlers" who have made a business out of monitoring new corporation filings, grabbing similar domain names, and then sending "congratulatory" letters to the new companies offering to sell them the domain names utilizing the name of their new company.

Another intellectual property expense is Web site development. As you build out your new company, you should simultaneously have a Web presence. There are many reasons to have a Web site even before your product is market ready. You may use the Web site to show partners, customers, and investors product research, features, and release dates. The site can reflect a positive corporate image to potential partners and investors. The longer your site is live on the Web, the more other sites will link to your site, and the better positioned it will be for search engine listings. You can find inexpensive Web site developers or use template

Web sites from companies such as Network Solutions, Intuit, or Word Press.

Some of the costs associated with building and hosting a Web site include the following:

1. Web development
2. Hosting the Web site
3. If you conduct commerce on the Web site, transactional costs for ecommerce merchant
4. Search engine optimization costs
5. Graphic art, designs, logos, stock photos

If your Web site will be more of a brochure than a Web application, then I would suggest inexpensive template-driven sites. These are do-it-yourself sites that look incredibly professional that you can launch for less than a few hundred dollars.

Budgeting for product development is critical. You must be organized and plan properly. Define precisely what you are developing and how long it will take. You need to set a schedule with defined milestones. Product development costs will vary based upon the type of product being developed. For instance, a manufactured product that depends upon additional component parts from outside sources is different than a technology product such as a web application. However, they both share in common the need to project and understand budget, timelines, cost of outside sources and additional other influences. This is critical. You will fall behind on your schedule if you don't understand this. You must hold your development team accountable for milestones, sticking to timelines, and budget adherence.

If you will be selling your product, then you need to budget for sales and marketing. This may include direct sales, sales representatives, advertising, and Web-based marketing. These items may be very expensive and inefficient.

Watch out. Monitor each marketing expense closely; otherwise, costs may get out of control quickly.

Before allocating marketing expenditures, you must understand the cost of acquisition of your customer. You must compare this to the lifetime value of your customer. I discussed this in great detail in Part I of this book, but here are some basics.

The cost of acquisition of a customer should be less than the "lifetime value" of the customer. In the early stages, your business model is fluid and adaptive. The cost variables such as lifetime value changes as your model changes. Be certain not to lose sight of the bottom line. Your bottom line is how much net income you create. The calculation of cost of acquisition versus lifetime value of a customer is critical to your bottom line.

Do the math. The cost of acquisition of one customer in an advertising campaign equals the cost of advertising plus the cost of sales force and marketing initiatives for that particular campaign. Divide that total cost by the total number of new customers acquired in that particular campaign.

For example, if it costs $1,000 to advertise online and it costs $1,000 to pay a sales person for a two-week campaign, then your total cost equals $2,000. If you acquire twenty new customers from this expenditure, then your cost of acquisition equals $2,000 divided by twenty (newly acquired customers). The cost of acquisition of a customer for that campaign equals $100 ($2,000 divided by twenty).

When the cost to acquire a customer is less than the lifetime value of the customer, the advertising campaign should be continued. If, however, the customer only represents $10 in profit with your company and it costs $100 to acquire that customer, than you have lost $90 per customer in that campaign. In that scenario, it is too expensive to advertise and acquire a customer. Conversely, if each customer generates $150 in profit and the cost of acquisition is $100, then your company nets $50. That is a much better business model.

The important concept to understand is "lifetime value" of the customer. The lifetime value of a customer validates the sales and marketing budget. The lifetime value, conservatively, assumes that your customer repeats purchases over a certain time period (a "lifetime"). You must know your customer's lifetime value to your company before creating any sales and marketing budget.

The lifetime value of a customer concept is universal to every business. It is the essence of "repeat customer." The prototype model for repeat business is a subscription business. The first year "x" amount of customers subscribe; the second year, half (1/2x) of subscribers renew; and the third year, half of those subscribers renew (1/4x). The lifetime value of this customer can be calculated as "net" or "gross." If it is calculated as net, it is bottom line profit per customer after costs. If it is calculated as a gross amount, it represents gross revenue before costs of goods sold. In the example above, net proceeds from the initial purchase plus 50 percent of the net proceeds of the first purchase (representing 50 percent of the customer's renewing for the second year subscription) plus 25 percent of the net proceeds of the first purchase (representing 50 percent of second-year subscribers renewing for the third-year subscription). This formula is representative of the lifetime value of a customer in a subscription-based business. If the subscription you were selling generated a net profit of $20, then the lifetime value would be $20 + $10 + $5 = $35. In this example, the customer's lifetime value is $35. The cost of acquisition for that customer should be less than $35 to be profitable.

Examples of some initial sales and marketing line item expenses:

1. Sales force salary or independent contractor sales
2. Commission on sales
3. Direct advertising sources and expenses
    a. Traditional media—TV, radio, and newspaper
    b. Internet advertising
        1. Pay per click
        2. Pay per call
        3. Behavioral marketing
        4. Affiliate marketing

Most companies book PR (public relations) as a separate expense from sales and marketing. They are two different expenses because they have two clearly different goals. Sales and marketing refers to generating customers or direct sales from these efforts. PR does not result in direct sales. PR results in corporate or product awareness. Although PR may translate into sales, its immediate impact and goal is to create awareness of the company or the product.

I am a big believer in PR, especially early in a company's development. You can generate significant "buzz" about your company without the expense of costly advertising.

I started PassportMD in 2004. PassportMD was one of the first personal health record companies. I started this company five years before President Obama started talking about electronic health records. When I first tested the business concept, I had no employees and no office. I decided to write a press release about the company. I wrote a release that had an angle. The angle is what gets the press to pick up your story. It is usually a human-interest angle. I wrote that I had a new way for seniors to protect their health when travelling away from home. At the time, this was novel. For a few hundred dollars, I sent the release over the wire. The AARP (American Association of Retired Persons) picked up the story and wrote about PassportMD in its national magazine. Additionally, I received coverage in several computer magazines and retirement magazines. As a result of one release and at a cost of just a few hundred dollars, PassportMD was covered in many newspapers and magazines. I could never have afforded that type of coverage through traditional advertising. I had a virtual phone with no office and no employees. My phone began to ring off the hook with customer inquiries.

There are two ways to approach PR. You can hire a PR firm or do it yourself through a Web site like prnewswire.com. Traditionally, PR is done through a PR firm, and often these firms are very expensive. PR firms may charge a monthly retainer and then charge based upon the "success" of the PR campaign. Every time a media outlet picks up the story, you get charged. The reach of the media outlet will determine the fee the PR firm charges. For example, if your company gets mentioned on national TV or in the *Wall Street Journal*, then it will cost you more than if your company gets mentioned in a local community newspaper. Some PR firms charge just a flat fee for a set project with a defined set of goals. In this instance, you may not get charged for each media "hit." You must negotiate that deal with the PR firm that you prefer.

I have approached PR both ways. A few years after I launched PassportMD, I hired nationally recognized celebrity spokesperson. She was the perfect spokesperson for our company. She was a mother of five and was committed to health and wellness. She was willing and able to talking about our product on national television.

However, to manage this, I had to hire a large PR firm. It was very expensive. It coordinated a radio and television satellite tour. It managed travel, hotel, and makeup for the celebrity. It coordinated schedules. It was successful and was able to land her on *Good Morning America* and many other nationally televised shows.

I have also done PR "the poor man's way." I prefer this. It is much simpler and can be just as effective. Start off by doing PR yourself. The advent of the Internet has enabled entrepreneurs to create a PR angle about their company and distribute the story themselves over the "wire." The "wire" is the term for an electronic distribution list that reaches news editors, organizations, and journalists. Journalists and editors may "pick up" the story. They write about it if it interests them and their audience. A release is short and easy to write. PR Newswire will review your PR release and will copy edit it at no extra charge before releasing it over the wire.

You should write the release yourself. I would suggest you copy the format of other PR releases from other companies. You can find these easily by going on Web sites and looking for links such as "In the News" or "Press Releases." It is very helpful to review your competitors' press releases. Remember your release must have an angle. It must not sound like an advertisement. You must have a human-interest side to your release. It should incorporate your product's information within the release. For example, do not write a release about your product being cheaper and more functional than competitors. Write a release that people with a certain problem can solve it by using your product.

Every business must be insured. You will have both personal and corporate liabilities. It is critical to understand these exposures and insure against them.

Each business will have different needs depending on the type of product the business sells. Here are the types of insurance coverage you will need when you first start your company:

1. You will need general liability insurance. This will protect you if someone is injured on your property.
2. Business interruption insurance will protect you in the event your business loses the ability to operate. This may be due to a variety of reasons, including loss of power. The office overhead policy pays payroll and other fixed business expenses. It enables you to keep your staff paid while you are unable to generate any revenue.
3. Depending on what you sell, you may also need product liability insurance to protect you from damages associated with use of your product.
4. Insurance to protect against breaches in personal information, someone "hacking" into your computer systems, or a rogue employee. You should discuss these policies with your insurance agent.
5. Workers' compensation insurance.
6. Director and officers' liability insurance (D&O). This insurance provides financial protection for the directors and officers of your company. This is like an errors and omissions policy for directors and officers.
7. Errors and omissions policy or malpractice policy, depending upon the type of services your company provides.

You will need a business office. Initially I used my medical practice as an office. It enabled me to determine if the business was viable and still maintain a practice. As each company grew out of my office space, I leased office space. Assume short-term leases only, and, whenever possible, take no more than twelve months. You should not be required to pay any more than first and last month's rent and a security deposit. Be certain that you do not sign any lease or contract personally. Always sign as a representative of the company with your title next to your signature.

You will need office equipment, supplies, and furniture.

Table 18 Initial office equipment requirements

1. Printers, computers, faxes, scanners

2. Phones (or phone system)

3. Furniture

4. Office file cabinets and bookcases

5. Networking equipment, routers, and servers

The office supplies include laser paper, pens, envelopes, stamps, paper clips, tape, scissors, whiteboard, and printer ink, to start. A whiteboard should be part of any entrepreneur's office. It fosters "brainstorming" and a creative environment. The staff should be encouraged to "step up" to the whiteboard and sketch out their ideas.

Printing gives your company a professional and consistent appearance. Logos and colors should remain consistent throughout your printed materials. Traditionally, printing was expensive. However, Internet sites offer commercial grade printing for much less. I recommend an online site called Vistaprint.com. It offers an easy, professional, and affordable online service.

Your greatest expense is payroll. This will make or break the company. Carefully choose the critical positions. Hire as many independent contractors as you can before hiring full-time employees. Be certain that your company is busy enough for full-time employees. As the owner of the company, you have personal liability to make payroll. Your employees can sue you personally for payroll. Be certain that you do not keep employees on the payroll if you cannot afford to pay them. Hire the absolute minimum number of employees to help you reach your next milestone. Resist the urge to hire additional staff until the business requires it. Remember, if you have employees, you must have workplace procedures, policies, and employee handbooks. Attorneys or payroll services can provide this either free or for a nominal extra charge.

These are some of the expenses that are essential to a start-up. Do not start your company until you have raised capital to cover three years of expenses. I made this mistake with my last company. I started PassportMD without enough capital. At the time I needed more investment in the company the economy had collapsed. Eventually, I did raise additional money from investors. However, given the desperate need, I diluted my ownership interest more than I preferred in order to secure the necessary capital.

Table 19. Common expense items and categories in the first two years of a business

1. Incorporation of your business

2. Intellectual property

3. Web site development and support

4. Product development

5. Sales and marketing expenses

6. PR (public relations) expenses

7. Insurance expenses

8. Office space

9. Office equipment and printing expenses

10. Employees and subcontractors

RAISING THE MONEY YOU NEED

If your company has no revenue, then you are a "start-up." You are in a conceptual stage. Your most likely source for funding will be "angel investors." Angel investors are usually friends, family, or wealthy individuals that get excited by the idea of a start-up. They have the capital to invest. They are very often familiar with you and want to see you succeed.

A "term sheet" is the legal document that you will receive from investors. It describes the terms that you have agreed to in exchange for the investment. A term sheet is nonbinding. This means that it is not a formal contract. Your best "terms" will be from angel investors. "Terms" refers to the amount of "dilution" and control you relinquish upon accepting an outside investment. Dilution means how much of your ownership gets shared amongst other investors. Raising money is selling stock in your company. You are bringing in co-owners and partners. You are "diluting" or reducing your percentage ownership of the company. Control refers to the number of voting seats designated to the investors on the board of directors.

Raising capital must be done according to state and federal laws. You cannot bypass this. There are strict laws that need to be followed even when raising money from angel investors. There is a need for full disclosures of the investment risk. This is critical. You will need the assistance of a corporate attorney to help you seek outside capital. The first capital raise for the company is referred to as "round one." Part of the legal work that is done is creating a "PPM" or private placement memorandum. The PPM will contain all the disclosures necessary to sell stock in your company. Lawyers will help you create a PPM, but much of the work you do yourself. At a minimum, the PPM will contain the business plan, the risks, the disclosures, the value of the company, and the value of the stock you are offering for sale.

Common questions from entrepreneurs are: How much stock should be sold to investors? How much ownership should be given up? What will be the resultant dilution to founders? These are the questions all entrepreneurs will ask of themselves. The answers lie in the valuation.

The valuation is determined by comparing your company to other companies in a similar business sector at a similar stage. Those are called "comps." You can find their value from a variety of sources on the Internet. You can find what other investors, public and private, have valued those companies at and try to correlate that to your company. Once you determine your valuation, you can then determine how much you can sell your stock for to investors. The "pre-money" valuation is the value of your company before you take investors. The "post-money" valuation is the value of the company after the investors' contribution. If you determine that your company is worth $2 million before any investors invest and you raised $1 million, then your "post-money valuation" would be $3 million. Investors would be buying into and owning one third, or 33 percent, of your company. In your PPM, the value of the shares of the company will be set from pre-money valuation. If you decide the company is worth $2 million, you would have two million shares issued at $1 per share. You may issue another one million shares for sale at $1 per share.

In your first round, you will need to decide a few other issues:

1. The minimum amount of shares you want to sell to any investor. Another way to look at this is the minimum dollar amount you will accept from any investor.
2. The term or amount of time you will give this round before closing it to additional investors.
3. Whether or not you can use the investment before you close or complete the round.
4. Whether or not you offer preferred shares (generally you reserve these for subsequent rounds with institutional investors (i.e., venture capitalists or VCs).

The other way to set a valuation for your company is less scientific. Ask yourself how much money you need. Then ask yourself how much ownership you are willing to give up. For example, if you need $1 million and you are willing to "give up" 50 percent of the company to raise that amount, then your pre-money valuation would be $1 million. Your post-money valuation would be $2 million. Another example would be if you need $2 million and are only willing to give up 33 percent of your company. In this scenario, your pre-money valuation may be $4 million. Your post money valuation would be $6 million. Because it is often difficult to find a truly comparable company to a start-up, valuations are somewhat arbitrary. They are related to how much money you raise and how much ownership you give up.

When I started Skinstore.com, it was in the middle of the dot-com boom. Valuations were sky high and based solely on an idea. We raised $2.5 million on a $6 million pre-money valuation. Four years ago when I started PassportMD, the capital markets were not as generous. I was forced to raise less capital with a lower valuation.

You should not wait to raise capital for your company. Founders may be concerned that they will be too diluted if they raise money too early. Don't fall into this trap. Get the money when you can. It is your lifeblood. If you have to give up more ownership to get it, do that. The capital will provide you with fuel to grow the company. The lack of capital will suffocate it.

Venture capital will be a better source for funding if you need $3 million or more in capital. Venture capitalists (VCs) are also called institutional investors. Be careful, as VCs are less forgiving than angels. They will have clauses that ensure that the business is being run they way they want. They may try to replace you or bring in additional board members to vote you out if the company is not being managed in the direction they prefer.

If you are the founder, then you must control the board. If you lose control of the board, then you will lose control of your company. The VCs may want to take the company in a different direction than you. It doesn't matter if you are successful or failing. In either scenario, with loss of board control, you lose. You must preserve your right to appoint the majority of the board members. Your term sheet outlines the terms agreed to by you and the investor. The term sheet should reflect how many board seats you offer to your investor.

There are many other "terms" found on a term sheet that should be reviewed carefully before signing.

Stock options may be included within the term sheet. The negotiation with stock options is whether or not the stock options come out of the pre-money valuation or post-money valuation. If the options come out of pre-money valuations, then the issuance of options further dilutes the founders.

Some term sheets may include a vesting plan for founders. This term is written so that the investors know that the founder will remain involved even after the founding event—in other words, not just leave after raising capital and taking money out of the business.

"Liquidation preferences" is the term for describing which shareholders get paid first from proceeds upon a sale, liquidation, or dissolution. Institutional investors will often purchase preferred shares. Preferred shares are in contrast to common shares. Preferred stockholders typically get paid first when there is a liquidation event. It is not uncommon for the institutional investor to also receive "participating preferred" shares. This means that participating preferred shareholders get cash upon liquidation for their preferred shares but also again for their percentage ownership of their common shares. This is commonly referred to as "double dipping." The term sheet will reflect that preferred shareholders participate with common shareholders on an as-converted basis.

Anti-dilution protection is the term used to protect the investors from being diluted upon subsequent fundraising rounds. This provision allows the investors to maintain the same initial ownership percentage if the company has to bring in additional future investors. That means that the founders take the hit on dilution rather than the institutional investors. This is commonly referred to as "full ratchet" provision. A weighted average basis will offer some protection to founders when included along with this provision.

A dividend provision may be included within the term sheet. This provision may specify a percentage dividend that investors receive when and if dividends are declared by the board. Dividends may or may not be cumulative. If they are cumulative, then they compound year after year.

A "no-shop" clause will be part of the term sheet. This keeps the founders from shopping the term sheet amongst other investor groups. Typically the no-shop period will be thirty to sixty days.

Another source of capital is from private equity firms. In general, private equity will not get involved in start-ups. They follow stringent investment guidelines. Private equity typically only invests in companies with significant revenue and cash flow.

The last source of funding to consider may be in the form of loans and bank lines. I would steer you away from these sources. They usually require personal guarantees. You should never do this with any start-up.

STAT CONSULT FROM JOHN IGOE, A CORPORATE ATTORNEY

Term sheets: Vesting of founder shares sounds ominous and unfair, but actually makes sense even for the founders if there is more than one founder. Investors want to know that key founders will remain involved in running the business. If a founder leaves before all of his shares are vested, the company will have a right to buy unvested shares at prices that often vary depending on whether the founder quit or is fired for cause, or is terminated without cause. Why should a founder who quits earn as much as a founder who sticks with the company and contributes to its appreciation?

Participating convertible preferred stock is usually structured to give investors a priority return equal to the amount invested (one times the amount, sometimes higher) plus a negotiated dividend rate, and then participation in the balance of sale proceeds with other common stockholders, as if the preferred stock was converted into common stock. Variations will cap participation at a fixed rate of return (e.g., five times), giving more upside to founders and other common stockholders.

Preemptive rights are a mechanism for permitting existing stockholders to participate in new financings in order to maintain their percentage interest in the company. These rights should be reserved for stockholders who qualify as "accredited investors" under securities laws to minimize the expense and delay of securities law compliance with disclosures for new financings.

Anti-dilution rights will not preserve an existing investor's then-current percentage interest in the company, but will give the investor the benefit of an adjustment taking into account the lower price per share of stock sold in a new financing. Full ratchet and weighted average are the two common formulas for anti-dilution rights, typically triggered by adjusting the conversion formula, giving the holders of convertible preferred stock the right to acquire more shares of common stock upon conversion of their preferred stock.

Other common terms include protective voting provisions and redemption rights. Even though a VC may not acquire a controlling position in your company, he or she will negotiate a laundry list of voting rights giving him or her veto power on major decisions like raising new capital, borrowing, changing the composition of the board of directors, and selling your company. This amounts to effective control in most scenarios. Redemption rights address VCs' concerns for an exit. After five years, a VC investor will have the right to give your company notice to repurchase his or her shares at a price equal to the greater of fair market value or, for example, the amount of their investment plus accrued dividends. Redemption rights are seldom exercised, but everyone knows when the trigger date is approaching. They create motivation for the board of directors to sell the company, find a way to buy out the investors, or, if everyone is on board with continuing to grow the company, to get a waiver or extension of the redemption rights.

VCs will do a lot of due diligence on you and your company. They tend to support experienced management teams versus great ideas. Assume that you will experience hard times ahead and that you will need to raise more capital in following rounds, and, accordingly, make sure you are comfortable with the VCs you select. Do your own due diligence and talk to CEOs of their portfolio companies before you sign that term sheet.

REALITY CHECK BEFORE YOU LAUNCH YOUR DREAM BUSINESS

With the first company I started, I was an expert in the field. Skinstore.com sold skin care products over the Internet. The company grew with little effort because I had relationships already with partners and vendors. I knew the business. I was not dependent upon any experts for help. As a dermatologist, I understood the value proposition to strategic partners and to end-users. Effortlessly I created significant relationships with partners and customers.

I started other companies. One was a robotic telepathology company, and another one was a personal health record company. Both of these businesses were highly technical. They required my dependence upon technicians and others. I could not analyze their work adequately. I was not enough of an expert to objectively judge their performance. I became frustrated with my reliance on others for objective analyses.

Before I consider any new business venture, I now ask myself if I am knowledgeable enough to write a book about that business. You should have that level of knowledge. Your business plan is like a book. It is a comprehensive document that reflects your expertise and understanding of the business.

I completed college and medical school in seven years. I completed an additional five years of residency training. Being an entrepreneur took a greater toll on me than those twelve years. Do not underestimate the challenges you will have in starting, running, and building a successful business.

Before launching a new career or a new business venture, ask yourself if you are qualified to write a book about that business. If you think that you would have to do a year of research beforehand, then you are starting against the odds. Choose a business in a field that you have expertise in from the start. Don't go into the restaurant business because you like to eat. Go into the restaurant business because you have the experience of working in the restaurant business.

THE TIME

If you think you can start a business and be a doctor, too, think again. I did it but I would warn against it. Even though there were successes, there were failures too. And there were costs, personal and financial. I could not devote enough time to meet both company's complete needs. A business is all-consuming. It will consume your creative energy, nervous energy, and physical energy. It is just too much to burn the candle at both ends. There are not many people like Steve Jobs that can be CEO at Apple and at Pixar simultaneously. If you want to start a successful business, then you should commit singularly to that business.

For the last ten years, I ran hectic between my practice and my start-ups. I made it work. I would start my day at 5 a.m. every day, seven days a week. I would work on the start-up until 9 a.m. I would see patients three and a half days a week. After a full day of patients or during lunch, I would schedule business meetings. When I was at home, I was either thinking about my patients or thinking about my start-up. Although I loved the excitement of having two businesses, the demands were great. There are exceptions but most often running both a practice and an entrepreneurial venture will be very challenging and exact its toll.

I think being an entrepreneur is in your genes. It is part of your makeup. It is the way your mind is programmed. You either "get it" or you don't. Entrepreneurs see opportunity in every aspect of life. This is an entrepreneur. The problem is that most entrepreneurs get more excited from the idea than they do about the execution of the idea. Most entrepreneurs consequently fail. Most entrepreneurs are visionaries. They get the big picture. They are not detail oriented. Successful entrepreneurs hire detail-oriented operational personnel to help manage the operational aspect of their business.

THE MANAGEMENT TEAM, BOARD OF DIRECTORS, AND ADVISORS

When is it the right time to hire a management team? A management team can be very expensive. Management salaries can drain your start-up capital. However, a good management team can make the difference between success and failure.

Initially, you do not need to hire a COO (chief operating officer). You can serve as both CEO and COO. You don't need to hire a CFO (chief financial officer). You can hire a part-time CFO or a controller. You should not hire a chief marketing officer until you have a product that is fully developed.

When the company has the revenue or sales to support management, then that is the right time. As good as a good management team may be, the wrong management team can be equally bad. It will increase your risk of failure. It can be expensive, distracting, and keep you from achieving your goals.

Don't hire an executive just because he or she is available. Research every option before hiring anyone. Research backgrounds extensively. If you hire the wrong person early on, it will stagnate your business. It will be costly, both financially and emotionally, to terminate him or her.

A laissez-faire attitude is a recipe for failure for any start-up. Start-ups are a constant battle between all the things that can go wrong and those that don't. A "weekend warrior" is not sufficient. Management must be 110% committed to deal with these issues. A part-time CEO cannot run a start-up. I founded a robotic telepathology company to help surgeons remotely connect with pathologists when performing cancer surgery. We were growing. My partner recruited a CEO for the company. It was a former partner of his from a prior business twenty years earlier. Let's call this person Joe. Joe accepted the position reluctantly. He was semi-retired and had done well in a business fifteen years prior. He was enjoying life as a consultant. Joe took the job because he felt obligated to my partner. Joe would come in to the office on a part-time basis. He would fly in from one of his many homes and run the company half-heartedly. However, the demands of any entrepreneurial venture are too great to hire a "part-time" CEO. This hire did not work out.

There is a lesson learned. I would only fill the critical management positions, such as CEO or COO, with a person that was hungry to succeed. A start-up requires a full-time commitment. It requires the sacrifice of most of a person's free time. If you hire someone that is unwilling or unable to commit eighteen hours a day, seven days a week, to run your company, then you may be hiring the wrong person.

THE BOARD OF DIRECTORS

Every company should form a board of directors. The purpose of the board is to help management run and govern the company without bias. The board is empowered by the bylaws of the corporation. Important decisions for the company, such as key personnel hires and budget, should be submitted to the board for approval.

If the company is approached for an acquisition, the board should evaluate the terms of the acquisition on behalf of the shareholders' interests. Typically the board is responsible for selecting and reviewing the performance of the CEO. In a privately held company, the board may have different responsibilities than those of a public company. The duties of the board as defined by corporate bylaws may vary amongst companies. I recommend creating a board of directors for any size company. The board will help management adhere to a budget and make tough decisions.

If you are the founder of the company, you want to ensure that your vision for the company remains yours and not the board's. Since the board may have all shareholders' interests at heart, you must protect your own interests. Sometimes the board may challenge or try to get rid of you as the founder. This occurs if your vision and theirs conflict.

You need to be prepared for certain problems with the board. This happens more often than you might expect. It is more common when your company is capitalized with venture or private equity capital. The way to protect yourself in advance with board conflicts is to make sure you have a majority of the seats on the board. As a founder, you should set up the company to preserve your right to designate a certain number of board seats. Ideally, you should have the right to appoint the majority of board seats. You can appoint board members that you think will be aligned with you in tough times. I would suggest that you never relinquish majority board control to any investor.

STAT CONSULT FROM JOHN IGOE, A CORPORATE ATTORNEY

All members of the board of directors, including the founder, have fiduciary duties under law to look out for the interests of all shareholders, not just the interests of the shareholders they might represent. Directors must obtain all material information relating to the operation of the business from management. Conflicts will arise with respect to any contracts between the company and a director or an affiliate of a director. In general, these transactions should be fair, and they should be approved by a majority of disinterested directors or by a majority of disinterested stockholders.

THE ADVISOR

The advisory board is distinct from the board of directors. The advisory board is created to give advice. Advisors typically have expertise or relationships that could help the company grow. The advisory board has no governing responsibility and does not vote on critical corporate matters. Sometimes the advisory board is created to give credence to the company for investment purposes. Founders will appoint well-known advisors in hopes of using their name to garner venture capital.

In 2010, the role of the advisory board as a tool to raise capital may be overrated. It was different in the early dot-com days. We assembled an incredible advisory board for Dermdex (another company I started). Dermdex was a B2B (business-to-business) marketplace we had created for dermatologists and plastic surgeons. The board consisted of world-famous thought leaders, prestigious Harvard Business

School faculty, and authoritative physicians. At that time, the board gave us instant credibility. The credibility helped us raise capital and forge significant partnerships.

Times have changed, and the value of the advisory board has been diluted by its overuse and ubiquitous presence. Savvy investors realize that they are often window dressing for a company.

I learned this with my last venture when I hired a celebrity spokesperson and recruited prestigious advisory board members. Although their presence was a great talking point, their true role as advisors was minimal. Also, advisory boards do not impress institutional investors such as VCs (venture capitalists) as they did before.

On the other hand, I have had a few advisors over the years that spent significant time with me. They have served as mentors. They taught me much without asking or wanting compensation. These types of advisor, if you are fortunate enough to find them, are rare. They want to help for the sake of helping. They want to see you succeed. Invite him or her to join your advisory board. In general, however, I would caution you, in the start up phase to not spend a disproportionate amount of your valuable resources (time and capital) on building the advisory board.

EVERYTHING IS NEGOTIABLE

I grew up playing poker. After thousands of games of poker, you learn how to read people. You see people act and react. You learn to hold your own. You learn to read your opponent and find your opponent's weakness. Poker is about folding at the right time. Fold too early and you will miss an opportunity to make money. Fold too late and you will have wasted an opportunity to save money. Business is like a poker game. Competitors bluff, competitors fold, and you win by competing. You must have nerves to play poker. You must have the nerves to compete in business.

Poker skills are needed to negotiate deals, hire key employees, and separate opportunities from dangers. It is a part of the hiring process as you negotiate a salary. Prospective employees will bluff you as you negotiate salaries with them. They will tell you that they make more than they make. They will try to make you believe that they have several offers on the table. You have to decide what to believe and what not to believe. You must make them an offer that is not too high but not too low either. If you are too low, you will lose them. If you are too high, then you will have paid unnecessarily. You must read the employees to see what they really want. You must see through your opponents' posturing. You must be able to read their eyes.

Every aspect of business is about negotiation. And every negotiation is like playing poker. Every deal must be negotiated from a position of strength, even if that position does not exist. You must create it. At times, you must be prepared to bluff to get the best results in negotiation. By bluffing I do not mean misrepresenting what you intend to deliver in the agreement. You should not do that. What I mean is that you must make the other party think that you do not need their company or the deal. Let them know you have other options or other companies waiting in the wings for the same deal. They must believe you are willing to walk away. Sometimes you have to walk away. If you walk away and you really do not have other options, that is bluffing. You must consider the consequences before the action. So, be careful. But, it is true, while in the midst of negotiation, the other party needs to believe that you don't need them. That is human nature and that is often the impetus for getting a deal done. However, I want to be clear, at the end of the day, for any agreement to work, both parties must be getting something they want. Do not misrepresent that. And, always deliver on your promises.

I remember cutting a marketing deal with the Microsoft Healthvault team early on with one of my companies. My vice president of business development and I were on the phone with four high-level Microsoft employees, including project managers and directors. We had a small office, a few employees, and no sales force. We were talking to them through a cell phone. We put the cell phone on speaker. We spoke to them from a position of strength. We negotiated a strategic partnership by telling them what our company could bring them. They agreed and we forged a nice working relationship together. I don't think we would have had a deal if they initially realized how small we really were.

The contract is the heart of every business. It does not matter the type of business. If you are successful, you will have negotiated a contract with a customer, vendor, or a strategic partner. It is the single most consistent item in any business. The contract transcends languages. It is what creates the value for your business. It is a handshake formalized by a signature. It is a business relationship defined by mutual agreement. The contract defines your costs when it is with a vendor and defines your profits when with a customer.

As an entrepreneur, you will be confronted with myriads of agreements and contracts. Every agreement has one thing in common: negotiation. Don't forget this. Negotiate every agreement before signing it. You must understand what you are signing, the implications, the opportunities, and the "way out." Negotiating is an art. It is the difference between success and failure. Do not assume anything is written in stone. It is just the opposite. Everything is written so that it can be negotiated. Ask for more than you expect and you will learn what it means to negotiate.

Table 20. Tips to follow before signing any agreement

1. Review the termination section and make sure you can always "terminate at any time without cause and without penalty."

2. Be certain that the jurisdiction for any disputes is always in your state.

3. Never sign any agreement personally (sign as a representative of the company).

4. Review the duration of the contract and the automatic renewal clause.

5. Understand your remedies in the event of disputes.

6. Review the use of your name, logos, press releases, and copyright intellectual property. Many partnerships will specify that they can use these materials, so be certain you agree. Be certain that you must approve any press releases that make use of any of the above-mentioned items.

7. Review the assumption of liabilities for any agreement you sign. Be certain to understand the hold-harmless clauses or indemnification clauses.

STAT CONSULT FROM JOHN IGOE, A CORPORATE ATTORNEY

Negotiations: Know what you want and need in any contract negotiation, but also do not lose sight of what the other party wants and needs. Bluffing and other poker techniques may work for some, but don't forget that an agreement has to give each party a fair chance to get what it wants and needs, or else the relationship will soon sour regardless of the terms of the agreement.

In tough negotiations, when the other side seems to have more leverage, you may have to be prepared to walk and, at the appropriate time, show that or do it in order to get the other side to act reasonably and close the deal.

Coordinate your negotiating strategy with your business attorney. Let the attorney handle discussions with the other side's attorney and bring in the business principals when necessary to break deadlocks on key business terms.

HOPE FOR THE BEST, PREPARE FOR THE WORST

Poker skills will help you when things go bad. And things can go really bad. I can speak from experience. These are the times that owning a company take its toll. The bad times can be cruel to you and your health. You must be prepared for the bad times as well as the good times. Business is indifferent to your personal well-being. Be warned. Be prepared. It is not fun.

The last company I founded put me to the test. Things were going well. We had a marketing deal with a very large, well-known technology company. We had a deal with a celebrity spokesperson to help us create product aware-ness. We had a pipeline of Web-based applications that were very cool and cutting edge. Medicare had selected us as one of a select group of vendors to participate in their personal health record study. The company had ten com-mitted and energetic employees. My investors, through a signed private placement memorandum (PPM), had signed on to invest a huge sum of money. The company had secured funding for the next eighteen months. We were in a position of strength, or so it seemed. I remember this well. It was a Friday evening. In the middle of one of the worst recessions in decades, I received an e-mail from a representative of the investor group. The e-mail revealed that the investor group was unable to continue to fund the company. It had run out of money. That was it. No warning. No notice.

I was stuck. I had payroll obligations and ongoing operational costs. I was personally on the hook for payroll. Payroll was costing $50,000 per month. The next day I called a staff meeting and let all my employees go. This was one of the hardest things I have ever had to do. I felt terrible.

I was juggling debt, operations, Web site, investors, corporate partners, and customers. All of them were up in the air, and all were about to come crashing down.

My only hope was to sell the company. I had built a fantastic, award-winning software platform. There was clearly value to the right buyer.

I found a suitor for our company. It liked our software and pursued us. However, selling a company is never easy. This was no exception. The negotiations were protracted. The deal should have closed in six weeks but it took six months. Posturing and legal reviews remained obstacles to closing. At one point I walked away from the deal. Be prepared for the worst. Read and understand every term of an acquisition agreement. Be careful.

I was fortunate and sold the company to an excellent company. I negotiated a settlement with every creditor. I paid off all debt. Despite the hardships, I would not trade the experience. I have fond memories of the company and find comfort in the software legacy that I created. It remains a viable software platform that still helps many people on the Internet. I am pleased about that.

When things go bad, remember, don't panic. Don't lose your poker face. Don't lose your edge. Don't lose your cool. I was put in a terrible, unexpected position. One day we had money, the next day we didn't. I was amazed at how patient creditors became. It was not fun. Although I could have walked away from all the debt, I didn't. I wanted to settle every debt with every creditor. I wanted to walk away holding my head up high. And I did.

If you find yourself in a similar position, take a deep breath. Realize it will work out eventually. Make sure your personal exposure is minimal or nonexistent. The following is my advice on how to handle this type of unfortunate situation. It is more common than you would think.

Let go of every employee immediately. Go to work on how you can settle with each creditor. You must be prepared to deal with that. Before you pay any creditor any amount owed, make sure he or she signs a release or settlement agreement. This protects you from creditors trying to collect more after you reach a settlement amount. Do not pay any ongoing bills. Hold them as long as possible. Contact all the vendors that you owe money to. Explain that your company is having cash-flow problems. Explain that you are doing everything you can to raise additional cash. Tell creditors you will pay them upon raising additional funds. Surprisingly, most creditors understood. If possible, make small payments to vendors to show good faith. Start selling off assets such as computers, furniture, or equipment. As you raise money from asset sales, use those funds to pay any personal liabilities. The most significant personal liabilities are payroll and payroll taxes. You must cover these in their entirety before any other debt.

The longer you wait to pay your creditors, the more frequently you will begin hearing from collection agencies. This was a new experience for me. A creditor turns over your bill to a collection agency. The collection agency plays "good cop, bad cop." It "understands" your situation and "wants to help." The agency becomes your "friend." It will tell you that any amount that you pay the agency will be used to pay off your debt. More importantly, the agency will explain, partial payments will keep it from turning over the case to attorneys. That is the threat. But be calm. The lawyers and the creditors know that if the company has no assets, the likelihood of collecting is low. Keep the collection agencies engaged for as long as possible. They will call you several times a week. They will threaten you. They will be aggressive. Hold off on paying them until you can afford to. And when you do pay them, pay them only a small amount. This will only last for so long. The collection agency will turn your account over to the lawyers. When the lawyers are involved, a new set of threats emerges. It is important to understand how the lawyers work so you can be prepared for this, too. The lawyers may get a percentage of what they collect. Or, they may have "purchased" the debt from the creditor. If they purchased the debt from the creditor, then they keep everything they collect. Either way you are now dealing with sharks. If the lawyer smells blood, he will attack. That means if he thinks there is money to be collected, he will sue you for it. They are professionals. Relax, take a deep breath, you still have time. They will hold off on suing you until the very last minute. Keep the dialogue going for as long as you can.

Hold firm. Negotiate with all your creditors. They are all prepared for the negotiation. The creditors just want to get paid. They will negotiate off a portion of your debt in exchange for complete settlement. Remember that you should pay off the personal liabilities first. Cover the remainder of creditor balances in order of importance to maintain the business operations.

If things go bad, stay calm. Approach liabilities in a systematic logical manner. Do not get emotional. Any business may fail. Most do. The point of this chapter is to help you handle yourself in this type of dire situation. Be prepared for the worst and hope for the best. Starting a business is very exciting. Closing a business can be very personal. It may be painful. Don't let it be. Remember business is business. Do not take it personally. Learn from the experience. Most businesses fail. Always have a contingency plan. Never burn any bridges.

I would recommend that you hire a corporate attorney to legally dissolve the company. This is money well spent. Attorneys will help you deal with the shareholders, assets, and liabilities of the company. If you are like most entrepreneurs, then this will not be the last company you create. Learn from your mistakes. Do not give up. Create a better company the next time. Success comes in many forms. As long as you keep trying, you will have success. Only if you stop trying will you have failed. So don't stop trying. Good luck.

CONCLUSION

It is not easy to be a physician and an entrepreneur. I believe that you have this trait in your genes. It is a departure from everything we learned in medical school. There are excellent examples of successful physicians that made the jump to business and made a fortune. These are the rare exceptions. I have lived in both worlds. I am excited and exhilarated by the business world. I enjoy the creative energy and the teamwork. I enjoy the art of negotiation and really enjoy cutting a great deal. However, it is not for the faint of heart. It is tedious and time consuming. An entrepreneur trades much of his free time for preoccupation with growing the business. In exchange, I have memories and experiences that will carry with me forever. I will never forget the excitement of seeing our spokesperson discuss our product on *Good Morning America*. I will always remember the first time flying to Seattle to meet with the Microsoft Healthvault team.

At the same time, as a physician, I have experienced the great joys of practicing medicine. I have patients that I will never forget. I have seen the good and bad in people. I have heard personal stories from my patients that make me cry and laugh. This is the invaluable experience of being a doctor. I am exhilarated when I perform a surgery, help solve a medical problem, or catch a serious cancer early.

Can a doctor wear both hats? Can a doctor be an entrepreneur and a caring physician? Yes, he can, and I did. You can, too. I hope through sharing my experiences in both worlds that I was able to enlighten you. I hope you can learn from my mistakes and get excited from my successes.

You can do whatever you set your mind to. Beware of the warnings, pitfalls, traps, and danger signs. Or, just ignore them, roll the dice and experience it yourself. It is exhilarating and rewarding when you create something new and different. It is exciting to create a team of hardworking, committed people selling your ideas. These are the rewards. Sometimes they are materially tangible, and other times they are intangible. Everyone has a different tolerance level for this. Some people should not risk the security and routine of seeing patients. The chaos and frenetic energy that are required for entrepreneurs are addicting but also can be overwhelming. You must ask yourself if you are up to the task before taking it on. Consider the worst and hope for the best.

Enjoy the ride.

Save the Date!

Earn CME hours and attend The Medical Entrepreneur Symposium March 29-April 1, 2012 at the Delray Beach Marriott Hotel in sunny south Florida.

RECEIVE CME CREDITS WHILE HEARING EXPERTS LECTURE ON EVERYTHING YOU NEED TO KNOW TO BE SUCCESSFUL IN PRACTICE AND AS A PHYSICIAN ENTREPRENEUR!

Register online at **www.TheMedicalEntrepreneur.com** and enter **coupon code TME2012** for additional 10% off registration fee.

SOURCES

Information from this book that was not my opinion was gathered from many sources. These sources include mostly Web sites and articles.

1. Skloff, Aaron. "Money Management Q&A." *Medical Economics Magazine*, June 4, 2010, p. 26.
2. http://www.hhs.gov/ocr/privacy/hipaa/understand-ing/summary/index.html
3. Chaudhari, R. "Will I receive stimulus money for adopt-ing an EHR." *Dermatology World*, September 2010.
4. Barry, Patricia. "A user's guide to health care reform." *AARP Bulletin*, May 2010, pp. 19–26.
5. http://www.aafp.org/online/en/home/practicemgt/mcareoptions.html
6. Sanders, Denise L., and Steven J. Kern. "HITECH act." *Medical Economics Magazine*, March 19, 2010, pp. 25–29.
7. "The 'meaningful use' regulation for electronic health records." http://www.NEJM.org, July 13, 2010, p. 1006114.

8. http://www.investopedia.com/terms/i/incomestatement.asp
9. http://www.investopedia.com/articles/04/031004.asp
10. http://www.investopedia.com/terms/r/retainedearnings.asp
11. http://www.incorporationmaster.com/
12. http://www.medicalpracticemanagement.com/medical_practice_management_consultant.html
13. http://www.florida-corporations-online.com/about-s-corporations.html
14. http://www.incorporationmaster.com/
15. http://www.caqh.org/
16. http://www.PracticeMgmt.com

Want to learn more from Dr. Hacker & leading experts on practice management and entrepreneurship?

Earn CME's and learn how to be a successful physician entrepreneur.

Attend The Medical Entrepreneur Symposium and ask Dr. Hacker and various business experts questions in person. Get invaluable business and practice advice! Meet and interview the vendors Dr. Hacker has used in his practice and businesses.

SAVE THE DATE!

March 29-April 1, 2012 at the Delray Beach Marriott Hotel in sunny south Florida. Register online to attend **The Medical Entrepreneur Symposium.** Enter **coupon code TME2012** to save an additional 10% off registration fee.

APPENDIX I: THE FIRST 25 STEPS TO TAKE WHEN SETTING UP YOUR PRACTICE

1. Create a name and purchase the domain name online.
2. Designate type of corporation.
3. Register corporation with state.
4. Trademark the practice name.
5. Apply for tax ID number (also known as FEIN number).
6. Apply for NPI (National Provider Identifier Number) number.
7. Apply for a medical license in the state you are going to practice in.
8. Apply for a DEA (Drug Enforcement Agency) license.
9. Apply for hospital privileges where you plan to practice
10. Start exploring managed care plans online.
11. Register with CAQH (Council for Affordable Quality Healthcare).
12. Register with PECOS (Internet-based Provider Enrollment, Chain, and Ownership System) for Medicare enrollment.
13. Make decision: a billing company or bill internally?
14. Start exploring electronic health record systems.
15. Make decision: practice management consultant?

16. Contract issues for employees and physician employees.
17. Create employment agreements and at-will employment offers.
18. Make decision: payroll internally or outsource to payroll service company?
19. Set up your office.
20. Select office space and initial office equipment needed.
21. Plan for advertising and marketing your practice.
22. Start a PR (public relations) campaign.
23. Understand HIPAA, Red Flags rule, and network security.
24. Set up QA (Quality Assurance) and QC (Quality Control logs) and lab logs.
25. Set up line of credit with local bank.

APPENDIX II: A LIST OF TABLES IN BOOK

ABOUT THE AUTHOR

After being selected as one of twelve students to enter medical school early through the prestigious Junior Honors Medical Program, I graduated from University of Florida medical school in 1989. I spent two years training in internal medicine at the University of Michigan in Ann Arbor. I completed my dermatology residency at the University of Florida in Gainesville in 1994. By the time I had completed all my training, I had published over twenty peer-reviewed medical articles in medical journals. I authored several textbook chapters in clinical medicine textbooks. As of the writing of this book, I have incorporated ten different businesses.

I started private practice in Boca Raton, Florida, in 1994. Within ten years of starting my practice, I had a patient database of over twenty-five thousand patients. The practice is highly efficient and successful.

At the end of 1996, I founded a company called Skinstore.com. I started this Internet company in a small corner of my house. I raised outside capital in an angel round from friends and family. This was at the beginning of the Internet boom. Skinstore was one of the first sites to sell physician-recommended skin care products (cosmeceuticals) online. Skinstore organically grew to one of the biggest online skincare sites. The company, under new management, has gone on to achieve cumulative lifetime revenues of over $200 million since inception.

In 2004, five years before President Obama started talking about electronic personal health records, I created a personal health record company called PassportMD. PassportMD was selected by Medicare for its personal health record pilot program. It was recognized as one of the top personal health record companies in 2008 by the leading electronic medical record industry trade show. I negotiated marketing and partnership deals with Microsoft Healthvault, and many other Fortune 500 companies as well as a nationally recognized celebrity spokesperson. I sold the company. Many people still use the award-winning health record software I created.

In this book I share the lessons learned from both the mistakes and successes I experienced.

THE MEDICAL ENTREPRENEUR
HOTLINE

If you are starting a medical practice or a new business and would like to ask the author questions or advice on any business topic, then visit www.TheMedicalEntrepreneur.com for details.

THE MEDICAL ENTREPRENEUR'S SYMPOSIUM

Attend the only symposium for doctors of its kind.

Earn CME credits and learn from Dr. Hacker and leading experts on how to be successful in your medical practice or entrepreneurial venture.

Join us at the Delray Beach Marriott Hotel in beautiful south Florida on **March 29-April 1, 2012.**

Register online at **www.TheMedicalEntrepreneur.com** and enter **coupon code TME2012** to receive an additional 10% off the registration fee.

ABOUT THE EXPERT CONTRIBUTORS

John Igoe, Corporate attorney

Mr. Igoe graduated from Brown University in 1976 and Boston College Law School in 1981. He learns the operations and businesses of his clients in depth in order to be in a position to render legal advice in the context of their goals. He has practiced law in Florida since 1983.

John's practice is focused on working with entrepreneurs and companies growing their businesses. His clients raise private equity from angel investors, venture capital funds, and other institutional investors. John also represents venture capital funds. He has worked in the venture capital arena since he started practicing law in 1981. He has advised start-up companies from inception to initial public offering and beyond. He has a strong reputation in Florida for his knowledge of venture capital transactions and securities law. He also works on complex corporate structuring, mergers and acquisitions, joint ventures, and general corporate matters.

Mr. Igoe currently practices corporate law with the firm of Edwards Angell Palmer & Dodge LLP, a national law firm with offices in Florida.

<u>Jeff Cohen,</u> Board certified health care attorney

Mr. Cohen is "AV" rated by Martindale Hubbell and is board certified by the Florida Bar as a specialist in health care law. He was named "Best Health Care Attorney" for Florida in 1995 at the Sixth Annual Medical Business Health Care Awards. He was selected by his peers as one of the Florida Legal Elite for 2008 and was recognized as such in *Florida Trend*'s July 2008 issue.

Mr. Cohen graduated from Florida State University (bachelor or arts cum laude, 1984) and Florida State University College of Law (juris doctor, 1987). His memberships include the Florida Bar (1987); Health Care Advisory Board (member); American Bar Association; the Florida Bar Health Law Section (executive committee member 1994–1997, chair of Managed Care Division (1993–1996), member of Health Care Law Certification Committee (2005–2008); American Health Lawyers Association; Florida Hospital Association; the Doctor's Advisory Network of the American Medical Association; and the American Society for Medical Association Counsel. He was a member of the Antitrust Advisory Committee to the Agency for Health Care Administration in 1993 and is an adjunct professor at Nova Southeastern University. He also provides consultant services to the publication *Medical Business*. Additionally, he is a member of the editorial boards for the "TIPS on Managed Care Newsletter," a publication of the IPA Association of America and *Medical Economics*. Moreover, Mr. Cohen is a certified arbitrator with the American Health Lawyers Association (AHLA). He is a frequent author and lecturer in the field of health care law.

Mr. Cohen is founder of the Florida Healthcare Law Firm, which specializes exclusively in health care legal matters and currently practices board-certified health care law in Delray Beach, Florida.

Howard M. Gitten, Intellectual property attorney

Mr. Gitten graduated from Case Western Reserve University School of Law and received his undergraduate degree from the University of Pennsylvania. He is an attorney in the West Palm Beach and Fort Lauderdale offices of Edwards Angell Palmer & Dodge, LLP. He brings a business perspective to technology issues, and his technology background to business issues. As a registered patent attorney, Howard has advised his clients in instituting cradle-to-grave IP regimes, from establishing rights to licensing IP and building joint development programs around a client's IP. In addition to protecting technology, Howard advises his clients when navigating the treacherous waters of other's property rights through the conducting of patent and trademark validity and infringement investigations. Howard is a past board member of the South Florida Technology Alliance, is a current board member of the MIT Enterprise Forum of South Florida, the founder of the MIT Fire Circle for entrepreneurs, and is a member of the first class of board-certified intellectual-property lawyers in the state of Florida.

Kenneth Edelman, Estate attorney

Mr. Edelman received his bachelor of arts degree from State University of New York at Stony Brook, his juris doctor degree from St. John's University School of Law, and his master of laws (LL.M.) in taxation from New York University School of Law.

Mr. Edelman's practice focuses on all areas of estate planning for a wide variety of clients, both domestic and international, and also includes work in the areas of prenuptial and postnuptial agreements, private foundations, probate, guardianships, shareholders' agreements, and other corporate work, as well as tax planning.

He has lectured widely on matters relating to estate planning and taxation.

Mr. Edelman formed his own firm, Kenneth Edelman, PA, based in Boca Raton, Florida, in July of 2005. He was formerly a partner with Arnstein & Lehr, LLP, a national firm based in Chicago, joining in 2003 to open the firm's new office in Boca Raton. From 1995 through 2003, he was a partner with Broad and Cassel, LLP, a Florida statewide law firm. He directed the firm's Trusts and Estates Department in Palm Beach County, representing clients for the firm's Boca Raton and West Palm Beach offices. From 2000 through 2005, Mr. Edelman was associated with the multinational Florida-based law firm of Greenberg Traurig. Prior to moving to Florida in 2000, Ken worked for Lazarow, Rettig & Sundel, a law firm with offices in New York City and California, primarily handling tax and estate planning matters for clients in the entertainment field.